Invisible

A Journey Through Adenomyosis and Endometriosis

Maria Yeager

ISBN: 9798351753102

Important notices:

The statements in this book are not intended to diagnose, treat, cure or prevent adenomyosis, endometriosis, or any other disease. The author accepts no responsibility for any illness or harm as a result of the use or misuse of the information described in this book.

The recommendations in this book are based on the author's own research of clinical studies. The author is not a physician. This book is not intended as a substitute for the medical advice of a physician. The reader should regularly consult with a physician in matters relating to her health and particularly with respect to any symptoms that may require diagnosis or medical attention.

Although the author and publisher have made every effort to ensure that the information in this book was correct at press time, the author and publisher do not assume and hereby disclaim any liability to any party for any loss, damage or disruption caused by errors or omissions, whether such errors or omissions result from negligence, accident, or any other cause.

Table of Contents

Preface

Adenomyosis – a word that I never heard until I had suffered from it for seventeen years.

A word that I had never heard until AFTER I had five surgeries, multiple invasive tests, and repeated blood draws.

A word that I never heard until AFTER I had been on numerous birth control pills, pain relievers, muscle relaxers, and many other medications.

A word that I had never heard until AFTER I had endured years of excruciating physical pain, extreme blood loss, and emotional distress.

A word that I never heard until AFTER it had significantly affected my quality of life for seventeen years.

This should never happen to another woman. EVER!

Adenomyosis is a disorder of the uterus. It is sometimes referred to as endometriosis interna, as it is similar to endometriosis. In this disorder, the innermost layer of the uterus (endometrium) invaginates into the muscular layer of the uterus (myometrium). In a normal uterus, the two layers are separate. When the endometrial tissue invades the myometrium, it can cause severe pain and excessive bleeding along with many other symptoms. Endometriosis, on the other hand, occurs when endometrial-like implants are found in the pelvis outside of the uterus. This disorder causes extreme pain, especially during menstruation (but not limited to menstruation).

This is my story.

I had both disorders which is not unusual at all. Years ago, I authored a short book on my struggle with adenomyosis. However, as time went by, I realized that I needed not only to discuss both disorders, but I also needed to tell my story in greater detail. I struggled as I drafted this book because it was hard to relive it, and it was hard to reveal many of my embarrassing symptoms. However, for the sake of the women who are struggling now or will struggle with these disorders in the future, I felt it was necessary to give the reader a truly clear picture of what these patients face daily.

The first half of this book is a detailed account of my personal battle with adenomyosis and endometriosis. In this part of the book, I have added additional small sections within the story as follows:

- **Medication facts**: These sections give more detailed information about the medications that were prescribed to me during the time that I dealt with adenomyosis and endometriosis.
- **Note**: These sections have additional information that may help the reader to better understand the story.
- **What we know now**: These sections include information about what we know today (2022). Some of these topics will be discussed in greater detail in the second half of the book. As you will note, some of the treatments that I received at the time are not advised now. This shows how little was known about this disorder at the time I went through it compared to what we know today. Although progress has been made, the progress is slow. We need to increase research and education at a much faster pace to help other women deal with these disorders.

The second half of this book discusses the following:

- **Basics of Adenomyosis and Endometriosis**: These sections include basics about the disorders that is known today. Please note that not all symptoms will be experienced by all adenomyosis and endometriosis patients. Some patients experience more pain, others experience heavier bleeding, and still others experience both. If you suffer from these symptoms and suspect that you may have one of these disorders, please visit a reputable physician who is an expert in treating endometriosis and/or adenomyosis.

- ♦ **Further information specific topics**:
  - Adhesions
  - Allergies
  - Aromatase Inhibitors
  - Bloating
  - Colorectal Resection
  - Dyspareunia (painful intercourse)
  - Endometrial Ablation
  - Estrogen Dominance
  - Excision surgery
  - Flaxseed
  - Fibrocystic Breast Disease
  - Gallbladder Disease
  - Gonadotropin-releasing Hormone Agonists (GnRHa)
  - Hysterectomy
  - Imaging
  - Infertility
  - In Vitro Fertilization
  - Irritable Bowel Syndrome
  - Leiomyomas (uterine fibroids)
  - Mirena
  - Platelet Aggregation and Mean Platelet Volume (MPV)
  - Progesterone, Vitamin D and Bone Health
  - Rectovaginal Endometriosis
  - Uterine Artery Embolization
  - Uterine Polyps
  - Xenoestrogens
- ♦ **Conclusion**

- ♦ **Appendix I** -Summary of the medications, tests, procedures, surgeries, OTC medications, etc. that I took/went through during the 17 years that I dealt with adenomyosis and endometriosis and during my post-hysterectomy years.
- ♦ **Appendix II -** Summary of abnormalities that have been seen in adenomyosis clinical studies. There are many clinical studies that have been done on these disorders, and many proteins, hormones, enzymes, etc. have been found to be abnormal in these studies. Many more studies need to be done to confirm these findings.
- ♦ **Appendix III** – Recommended treatment facilities.
- ♦ **Appendix IV -** Recommended books.
- ♦ **Acronyms** – if the reader becomes confused by the acronyms used in this book, he/she can refer to this section. I realize that medical acronyms can become very confusing for those who are not scientists!
- ♦ **Definition of terms**: I have added this section in case the reader becomes confused with any of the terms in this book. If the reader is new to learning about adenomyosis, some of these medical terms may be quite confusing. Please refer to this section if you come across a word in the book that you don't understand.
- ♦ **References**
- ♦ **Index**
- ♦ **About the Author**

As you read this book, you may wonder why I discuss certain topics because they may not seem related to adenomyosis or endometriosis at all. However, by the end of the book, you will come to understand why I discuss these topics. For now, just know that there is a reason for everything that I discuss in this book.

I hope that the reader will not only gain insight into what an adenomyosis and endometriosis patient must deal with daily, but

that he/she will also gain knowledge on how to support women
who are affected by these disorders.

Blessings,

Maria

Part I – My Story

The Early Years

"Wait...I have more questions," I said.

"Hurry up. I have lots of other naked women waiting on me," my gynecologist responded as she headed for the door.

I wanted to ask her about my pain - my severe, unrelenting pain - but she seemed like she was bothered. It seemed like she was just too busy for my "minor" issues.

I felt ignored. I felt invisible.

It was a very lonely time in my life.

This is adenomyosis and endometriosis. This is what these uterine disorders put us through – those of us unlucky enough to be plagued by them.

Growing up in a small suburb of Cincinnati, Ohio, I had very few health problems. Of course, I had the occasional cold or flu, but other than that, I was a healthy, active, and happy child. The only real issue I had as a child was an occasional outbreak of itchy eczema on my waist that my mom treated with some hydrocortisone cream.

My menstrual cycles started when I was 14 years old which is normal by any measure. However, painful menstruation for me began with my very first period. I was selected to play Mary in the 8th grade production of a Christmas show at my Catholic grade school. As I stood on the altar dressed up as Mary and holding a little baby, I started to feel sick. My stomach hurt as I rocked the little baby back and forth, hoping that he didn't cry until after the show was over. By the time I left the altar, my stomach was really hurting, and I wondered if I had food poisoning. That evening, after the show, my family gathered at my aunt's house for our Christmas Eve celebration.

I sat down and was quiet because I felt sick. I told my mom that I didn't feel well, and she just told me to rest. When dinner was served, I ate, but my appetite wasn't good because my stomach hurt. After dinner, I went to the bathroom. I was shocked when I found a great deal of blood in my underwear.

"Mom," I called out the bathroom door. She quickly responded.

"What's the matter?" she asked as she walked into the bathroom. I showed her my underwear.

"Oh, you started your period!" she exclaimed. My aunt knocked on the door, and my mom cracked the door to talk to her.

"Do you have a maxi pad?" my mom asked my aunt.

"Oh, sure," she responded. A few minutes later, she returned. I put on my first maxi pad that night, the first of who knows how many I would have to wear in my life.

"Is this why my stomach hurts?" I asked my mom.

"Yes," she replied. "It's normal to have cramping with your period. I'll get you some aspirin. That will help."

After I took the aspirin, I felt much better.

***

As my teen years progressed, I noticed that my periods were quite painful, lasting up to ten days, and were very heavy. There were times during those years when I was in so much pain that I could barely walk. I was given NSAIDS (Motrin) to help control the pain, and this did help, but I remember thinking that I seemed to have more problems with my cycle than my other friends.

My family did have a history of some health issues involving the reproductive organs. My maternal grandmother was diagnosed with breast cancer in her late 30s, and she passed away from it in 1940 at the age of 41. Later in life, her sister also died of breast cancer, but this could be attributed to age. Other family members suffered from heavy and painful menstruation, large blood clots during menstruation, uterine fibroids, depression, severe mood swings, and even nausea/vomiting during menstruation.

During high school, there were several times I had to come home from school due to severe pain. I usually took Motrin and slept most of the day. I specifically remember having horrible cramping and very heavy bleeding one summer day when I was about 16 years old. Some of my friends and my brother wanted to go to a movie, and I really wanted to go, but I was in terrible pain. I took a Motrin during the morning hoping that it would help the cramping in time for me to be able to go to the movie. I curled up in a fetal position on the couch and hoped that the cramps would pass. The cramps were intense, and I dripped with sweat and felt nauseated. I was so pale that I looked like a ghost. When it was time to go to the movie, I decided to go even though I was still in pain. For the first half of the movie, I was in such pain that I really didn't enjoy myself at all, but the cramps finally started to ease up during the second half. By the time I left, the pain had relented, but it left me completely exhausted.

In college, I had some heavy periods and some intense menstrual cramps at times, but some months were OK. Other girls on my floor had some bad months as well, so I just thought it was normal. I was jealous of the girls that seemed to just breeze through their periods. One of my college roommates had the occasional bad period. I specifically remember one day when I returned to my dorm room only to find my roommate in her bed with severe cramps, and she had turned the thermostat up in the room so high that I could hardly breathe when I walked in! But I completely understood. I had times during my period when I was freezing cold and when I laid under multiple blankets and a comforter to keep warm.

In my freshman year, after a particularly bad period, I decided to go to the infirmary on campus to discuss my period problems with a doctor. When she came into the room, she asked me about all of my symptoms, and I gave her a detailed account of my gynecological issues.

"Have you ever had a pelvic exam?" she asked.

"No," I responded.

"OK, I think we need to do that." She walked over to a cabinet, pulled out a blue paper-like sheet, and handed it to me.

"Take off your pants and underwear and cover yourself with this. I will be back in a few minutes."

I did as she said and waited. A few minutes later, there was a knock on the door.

"Are you ready?" she asked through a crack in the door.

"Yes," I replied.

She entered the room and pulled a stool up to the bottom of the exam table. She told me to lay back, and she lifted the blue paper that covered me. I immediately felt uncomfortable. This woman's face was looking directly at my crotch. I knew I wasn't going to like this too much, and anxiety kicked in.

"OK, Maria, I am going to insert this into your vagina." She showed me this thing that looked like a duck's beak. "This will help me to visualize your cervix to see if there are any abnormalities. Ready?"

"Yes," I said quietly.

As she placed this "duck's beak" into my vagina, I felt immediate, searing pain. Between having her face in my crotch area and the pain that I felt, I began to breathe heavily. The anxiety took over completely. Things around me became blurry. The next thing I knew, the doctor was repeating my name repeatedly.

"Maria, Maria, can you hear me? Maria? Maria?" I realized that the doctor was standing next to me.

"Yes," I finally responded, realizing that I had not been coherent.

"Breathe normally. Try to slow down your breathing."

"What happened?" I asked.

"You are hyperventilating," she responded. "Slow down your breathing." She helped me until I breathed normally again.

"Are you OK now?" she asked.

"I think so," I responded.

She returned to the bottom of the table and continued with the exam as I focused on my breathing.

"OK, we are done," she said.

"I think I need to go to the bathroom," I said.

"OK, sit up for a minute."

I sat up, still feeling a bit dizzy from my experience.

"Do you feel alright?"

"Yes, I think so," I responded even though I was still dizzy.

"OK, let me help you to the bathroom."

As I walked to the bathroom, I started to see stars. Being as young as I was at the time, I didn't want to look weak, so I told the doctor I was fine. However, once she left, I almost passed out. Everything around me turned black. I grabbed onto the sink and wall, leaned over, and took in some deep breaths. My symptoms slowly subsided, and I managed to go to the bathroom. I was able to make it back to the exam table where I sat down and waited for her to return.

"I am NEVER going to have that done again!" I told myself.

The doctor returned and asked again how I was feeling.

"I'm OK," I said.

"It's not a pleasant test, especially the first time," she said.

"You're not kidding," I thought to myself as she looked at my chart.

"Well, I don't see anything abnormal on your exam. Ibuprofen is probably the best thing to take for pain. Some women just have heavier and more painful periods than other women."

All I knew at that moment is that I wanted to leave. I really didn't care what the doctor said. I just wanted out, and I never wanted to have that exam again. Little did I know that was the first pelvic exam out of innumerable ones that I would have in my life.

Allergies

My first experience with allergies occurred when I was about 8 or 9 years old. The sides of my abdomen would break out in an itchy red rash that would weep and crust over. The itchiness was almost unbearable at times. My mom took me to the doctor, and he diagnosed me with eczema. I was given some cream to put on it which helped to heal it. It recurred multiple times during the next ten years or so, but eventually it just went away until I entered menopause. I now have occasional outbreaks for unknown reasons.

In my teenage years, I developed some significant respiratory allergies. My grandparents love animals and had lots of cats. When I visited them, my eyes became extremely itchy and red within a few minutes of being around the cats, and I sneezed like crazy. My brother reacted in a similar fashion. We were told that my maternal grandmother had bad allergies and asthma, so we all just shrugged it off, thinking it was "just in our genes." If we were really uncomfortable, we would take a Benadryl and things would calm down a bit.

In addition to the cat allergy, I had some antibiotic allergies. My mom became aware of my penicillin allergy when I was very young (I broke out in a rash), and I became extremely ill after taking sulfa antibiotics for a urinary tract infection in my early teens. Seasonal allergies really started to affect me in my late teens. In college, I was so miserable in spring that I would sit in class while holding a tissue to my nose to catch the constant nasal drippage. If I didn't have a tissue, it was awful as I would sniff every few seconds so I would not drip all over my paper and book.

When I was a teenager, I decided to get my ears pierced. I was so excited to finally do this, and I was even more excited to go out and buy some fashionable earrings so I could look "cool." The original studs didn't cause me any trouble because they were gold; however, once I started to wear the cheaper earrings, my ears started to break out in an intensely itchy rash. The rash was all over my earlobe and even on part of my face and neck. I eventually had to stop wearing them. I didn't realize it at the time, but it was the nickel that was causing the reaction.

Years later, I tried piercing my ears again, but the same thing happened. As soon as I started using the nickel-plated earrings, the rash came back full force. Even some of the cheap bracelets that I wore resulted in that same itchy rash on my wrist.

After college, I finally addressed the allergy issue and visited an allergist. After testing, I found out that I had terrible allergies to all kinds of trees. This would explain why I was so miserable in the spring when all the trees bloomed. In addition, I was moderately allergic to cats, and I had a strong allergic reaction to ragweed. I decided to move ahead with allergy shots which ended up working quite well for me. After going through years of shots, my allergies improved quite a bit, but they never went away completely.

> ***What we know today***: **Endometriosis and adenomyosis have been shown to possibly be an autoimmune disorder. In addition, asthma and other allergic conditions have been shown in clinical studies to be linked to aberrant hormone levels, and nickel allergy has also been linked to these disorders. This will be discussed at length later in this book.**

Appendicitis

In the summer of 1985 while on summer break from college, I woke up one night with tremendous abdominal pain and nausea. I had just worked a ten hour shift the day before, and I felt fine during work. Luckily, I was at home and not at school when I became ill. I thought I had the stomach flu at first, but the abdominal pain became so severe that I began to think that something much worse was happening to me. I vomited for several hours, and then I started to have dry heaves. The abdominal pain was intense. I tried to sleep. As I looked at my clock, I would close my eyes and fall asleep only to realize when I woke up that I had only been asleep for a few minutes. When the dry heaving finally slowed down, my mom made me some soup and tried to get me to eat some of it. I tried, but it was as if there was something in my throat preventing me from swallowing. I absolutely could not swallow one sip of that soup. I gave up went to sleep on the couch. I slept about 45 minutes, the most I had slept in about 24 hours, but when I woke up, I had such severe abdominal pain that I could barely stand. My mom decided to call the doctor, and he told her to give me some Mylanta. He also told her that if she didn't notice notable improvement in me over the next couple of hours, she needed to take me to the emergency room. Finally, that evening, she did decide to drive me to the hospital. I have spotty memories of what happened from this point forward. The only memory that I have of my trip to the hospital was holding a pillow to my stomach and looking up at my mom as she drove. I now think I was blacking out. I had to rely on my mom's recollection of what happened from that point forward.

We arrived at the hospital, and I was taken back for the examination. The emergency room doctor believed that I had a bad case of the stomach flu. I was severely dehydrated, so I was put on an IV for rehydration. I was given a milky drink, similar to Mylanta, that was supposed to settle my stomach, but about fifteen minutes after drinking it, I vomited. I found out later that the doctor had ordered a tranquilizer to be added to my IV, so I had been sedated. When I finished receiving fluids through the IV, the doctor once again came in and, according to my mom, he was overly concerned about my condition. He decided to examine me one more time before I left to go home. This time, he pressed on the right side of my abdomen, and I jumped. When this happened, he immediately ordered a complete blood count. When the test came back with an extremely elevated white blood cell count, the course of my treatment changed very quickly. The right-sided pain along with the high white blood cell count suggested appendicitis. The ER doctor called my uncle who was a surgeon at that same hospital, and he immediately came in. I remember my uncle standing over top of me as he tried to talk to me.

"Maria, do you hear me?"

Barely coherent, I responded, "Yes."

"You have acute appendicitis, and we have to operate."

"When?" I asked.

"Right now," he replied.

That was about 2 a.m. I was wheeled into surgery at around 3 a.m.

When I woke up from surgery, I was shocked to find out that my appendix had ruptured and was covered in gangrene. Apparently, I had been suffering from appendicitis for a while. This explained my weird stomach symptoms that had occurred the previous semester at college. I remember one night during that semester when I suddenly became extremely nauseated. Oddly, I felt like I couldn't breathe. It was freezing cold outside, but I opened all of the windows in my room to get fresh air. When my roommate came into the room, it was so cold, and I apologized profusely. I explained to her what was happening to me, and she was so understanding. Suddenly, the symptoms disappeared as quickly as they appeared. It was one of the strangest things I had ever experienced.

After surgery, my mom told me that my uncle said it was probably the worst appendix he had ever seen, and he said that I was going to be sick for an exceptionally long time.

The next morning, I remember being visited by nurses from other floors and even the pathologist who examined my ruptured appendix. They were amazed that I actually walked into the hospital the previous night.

"You should have come in here unconscious and by ambulance! How in the world did you walk in here with an appendix in that kind of shape?"

"Well, I don't remember walking in if that tells you anything," I responded while chuckling.

I recovered quicker than most people expected. In fact, I was back to work three weeks after surgery. I vividly remember the horrible abdominal pain associated with this ruptured appendix, and I will never forget what my uncle said to me after surgery:

"Maria, if you ever have pain like that again, get yourself to a hospital immediately! This could have killed you!"

This one statement has always stayed prominent in my mind, and it ended up playing a significant role in what I was about to go through.

Genetic Translocation

I received my B.S. degree in Microbiology; however, my favorite subject in college was genetics. I worked for several years as a microbiologist, but when the chance to work in a genetics lab was offered to me, I took it. I was so intrigued and excited to work in genetics and chromosome analysis.

During my first few weeks, my boss asked me if I wanted to have a chromosome analysis done on myself. I jumped at the chance to have this done. I wanted to see what my own chromosomes looked like. I did not expect to see any abnormalities, and I was stunned when the results showed that I had a genetic translocation.

Genetic translocations are actually not that uncommon. A translocation can be balanced or unbalanced. A balanced translocation results in a karyotype with the right amount of genetic material present, but it is just located in the wrong place in the karyotype. This results in a normal phenotype meaning that the person appears normal. In these cases, there is an increased risk of miscarriage or abnormalities in future pregnancies. An unbalanced translocation is a karyotype that has either too much or too little genetic material present. Unbalanced translocations result in either an abnormal phenotype or an increased risk of miscarriage, depending on the amount of genetic material involved.

27

I have a balanced translocation. It involves chromosomes 1 and 15. Since the translocation was large, my boss explained to me that if I got pregnant, I faced a miscarriage risk of about 50% in theory; however, in cases like this, the reported risk is actually a bit lower than that. I also had about a 25% chance of the fetus having a balanced translocation (just like me), and about a 25% chance of the fetus having normal chromosomes.

I immediately thought of my mom because she had several miscarriages. I knew that this translocation could have just happened in me (de novo), or it could have been passed down to me from one of my parents. I asked my boss if she could test my parents, and she agreed to do so. I went home that day and explained all of this to my parents, and they agreed to the test.

It turns out that my mom carries this translocation. In addition, my siblings were tested. My sister has the translocation, but my brother has normal chromosomes. My mom's reproductive history made sense. We now knew why she lost some of her pregnancies.

I was happy to be able to give my parents this information as it answered questions that they had, but it was hard for me to get this same information. I was now facing an approximately 40 to 50% chance of miscarriage in my future pregnancies.

South Carolina (1990-1997)

1990

"Yet over two decades of my practice, it has become clear to me that healing cannot occur for women until we have critically examined and changed some of the beliefs and assumptions that we all unconsciously inherit and internalize from our culture."

-Christiane Northrup, MD, from her book, Women's Bodies, Women's Wisdom

The worst part of my health journey began in 1990. I was 26 years old. There were times in high school where I had to come home from school, take Motrin, and sleep the rest of the day away due to strong menstrual cramps. There were times when I was tired from all the blood loss. But those days pale in comparison to what was about to happen.

On a Friday night after a date with my boyfriend, I woke up at about 4 a.m. to waves of contraction-like pain that started in the small of my back and moved into my lower pelvis. These waves of severe pain came every two to three minutes. I had just finished my period, but I was still spotting. The pain was so intense that I could barely breathe. Nausea quickly set in, so I tried to get up to go to the bathroom thinking I was going to vomit. A wave of pain hit me again which caused me to drop to the floor. I literally crawled to the bathroom.

Once in the bathroom, I pulled myself up to a standing position by holding onto the sink. After turning on the light, I squinted into the bathroom mirror and noticed that I was white as a ghost. Another wave of pain hit me, and I doubled over, still holding onto the side of the sink.

I looked in the mirror again. Beads of sweat dripped down the sides of my face. I felt nauseated. I lifted the toilet seat in case I needed to vomit. As I grabbed a washcloth to wipe my face, another wave of pain hit me. This time, I became so lightheaded that I saw stars. I thought I was going to faint, so I steadied myself away from the sink in case I fell, one hand on the side of the sink, and one hand on the wall.

I thought maybe I had food poisoning. I felt like I needed to defecate, so I sat down on the toilet. I pushed, but nothing happened. I pushed harder. Nothing. I noticed that my abdomen was enlarged. It was pooched out as if I was pregnant. I stood up, and another wave of pain pushed across my abdomen. I fell to the floor.

I didn't know what to do. Each time the contraction occurred, I rocked back and forth on all fours and tried to breathe slowly. That's all I could do. I had no idea what was happening to me, and I couldn't do anything to control it. At one point, I tried to defecate again, but I couldn't. The nausea was unrelenting. Although I never actually vomited, I felt very close to doing so multiple times, my head curled over the toilet.

"Was this somehow connected to my appendicitis?" I thought. I remembered what my uncle told me:

> *"Maria, if you ever have pain like that again, get yourself to a hospital IMMEDIATELY! This could have killed you."*

Now, here I was, in WORSE pain than what I remembered during my ruptured appendix ordeal.

I managed to get to the phone to call my mom, and she came to my apartment immediately. When I opened the door to my apartment, I was doubled over in pain, white as a ghost, and sweating profusely. She was shocked to see me in that condition.

"What happened?" she asked. Her furrowed brow showed her extreme concern.

"I don't know," I replied, my hands clutching my abdomen.

"I'm taking you to the hospital."

"I'm in severe pain and I don't think I can make it to the car."

"You can do it. Come on. You can make it," she responded as she grabbed my purse. I held onto her arm and tried to control my breathing as we slowly walked to the car.

Once we made it inside the ER, I told my mom that I was going to the bathroom. I felt the urge to defecate, and this time, the urge was more forceful. I had a huge bout of diarrhea. There was a sense of relief after this happened, and the pain seemed to slightly improve afterwards. However, even with improvement, I still was in a great deal of pain.

We were finally called back to a room. When the ER physician entered the room to examine me, I was curled up on the stretcher in the fetal position. After his examination, he concluded that I had food poisoning. Since I was in so much pain, he gave me a pain shot which helped tremendously. I was sent home where I spent the rest of the day in bed asleep, completely exhausted from this horrendous experience.

After I recovered, I didn't think much more about what happened. I occasionally thought about the degree of pain that I endured as I had never felt anything like it before. I just hoped that it would never happen to me again, but that hope quickly dissipated about a year later when the exact same thing happened again.

1991

"That's one of the main reasons endometriosis gets undetected, because the symptoms are not understood well by the primary practitioners. They are referred to a GI doctor. And after many, many endoscopies and colonoscopies, patient still doesn't know where the problem is."

-Dr. Tamer Seckin

I woke up in the middle of the night with that same severe and debilitating pain that had attacked me on that fateful Friday night in 1990. Once again, this occurred right at the end of my period. The pain was unbearable, and again, the pain occurred in the small of my back and moved into my lower pelvis. I crawled to the bathroom and laid there, crying, in the fetal position. Sweat dripped own my face, and my shirt was soaked. Every time I tried to stand up, I felt like I was going to pass out. Fear and confusion overtook me. What was happening to me?

I kept trying to have a bowel movement, but nothing happened. I felt this horrendous need to push. The pain kept coming in waves, and all I knew was that the pain was worse than the ruptured appendix. I was convinced something was seriously wrong. I thought the physician at the ER must have missed it. Eventually, I had another bout of diarrhea, and the pain eventually subsided. The next day, I made an appointment to see a general practitioner.

During that appointment, I explained that this was the second episode of severe abdominal pain in the past two years, and I made sure he knew that both times occurred at the end of my period.

"I am thinking that this must be related to my menstrual cycle because both times, the attack occurred just as my period was ending. I was just spotting."

"Hmm," he responded. "Well, it also could just be a virus or something you ate, and it just happened to occur at the same time in your cycle."

I thought a minute. "Well, I guess that's possible."

"There's something else to consider," he continued. "There is something called irritable bowel syndrome, also called IBS."

"What's that?" I asked.

"Well, the symptoms are alternating constipation and diarrhea. It's a functional disorder of the intestinal tract."

"That's what is happening to me," I responded. "I get really bad constipation, and the pain ends when I have diarrhea."

"It's something to keep in mind," he responded. "The problem is that it's a diagnosis of exclusion. That means that we have to rule out all other causes of your symptoms before we can diagnose you with that."

"Oh," I said. "So, what do I do now?"

"Well, I can refer you to a gastroenterologist for further testing. This would probably start with a colonoscopy."

I frowned at this. I was scared to death of having some doctor put a tube up my rectum. "That kind of scares me," I responded.

"Well, we can wait and see if it happens again. In the meantime, I would suggest drinking plenty of water and increasing your fiber intake."

"Like eating more vegetables?"

"Yes, that's good, and also more fruit. But you may want to include Metamucil too. Once a day."

"Doesn't that stuff taste bad?"

"No, it's not bad at all. It's orange flavored, so it tastes like an orange fruit drink. Not bad at all."

"Oh, OK," I responded.

After that appointment, I picked up the Metamucil and went home. My general practitioner was right – the Metamucil wasn't bad at all. I started to take it every morning before work. However, the attacks didn't stop, and in fact they became more frequent.

> ***Note***: **IBS, or irritable bowel syndrome, is a functional disorder of the large intestine. It is also referred to as spastic colon.**

> ***What we know today***: **It is now known that endometriosis and adenomyosis are frequently misdiagnosed as IBS. Much more detail on this topic is addressed later in this book.**

The attacks continued and started to become more frequent. In addition to the attacks occurring at the end of my period, I noticed that my stomach would swell just before the pain started – that was the red flag that an attack was imminent.

> ***Note***: **Bloating is seen in over 80 percent of endometriosis patients and is commonly referred to as "endo belly". This topic is discussed in greater detail later in this book.**

I became more convinced that this was somehow related to my menstrual cycle. Additionally, I noticed that the pain affected my left side more than my right side. I started to use quite a bit of ibuprofen just to get through my period.

Menstruation for me was usually around 10 days or so at this point, and I had about 2-3 days of super heavy bleeding. I was working at the time, and it was exceedingly difficult for me to stop what I was doing in the lab because tests are timed. Many times, I knew I needed to go to the bathroom and change my maxi pad, but I could not do that because I was in the middle of a timed procedure. I could feel the gush of blood, but I could not stop. When I finally was able to go to the bathroom, I almost always bled onto my underwear. I remember several times where I walked to the bathroom very carefully, with my legs pushed together walking in small steps for fear that blood would drip down my legs. There were also times when I felt a gush of blood while driving home, and when I finally arrived home, there was some blood on my car seat. I learned that during my period, it was necessary to wear black pants just in case I bled onto my clothes. I would also wear either a long top or a long sweater just to make sure that any blood wouldn't show up on my pants if I leaked. Wearing anything white during my period was completely out of the question.

In addition to all the pain and heavy bleeding, I suffered from fairly severe PMS. Trivial things that didn't bother me during other times of the month became huge problems during PMS. My patience didn't exist during PMS – I would get bothered at the smallest things, such as someone in a car taking too much time to move after a light turned green or if someone drove below the speed limit. I would find myself cussing them out. I would occasionally have periods where I would cry over something small like not being able to find a matching sock or not being able to find my keys.

Around this time, I started to suffer from extremely sore breasts prior to and during my period. At first, I did not think much of it as I thought it had something to do with PMS. But after about a year of this achy pain, I started to worry because my grandmother died of breast cancer. I was not sure what to do, so I made an appointment with a gynecologist to ask him about this. He told me all about fibrocystic breast disease.

> ***Note:*** **Fibrocystic breast disease refers to painful, swollen, and lumpy breasts.**

"Yes, you have very lumpy breasts," he commented during the breast exam.

Once he finished the exam, he recommended that I have a mammogram.

"Since you have a family history of breast cancer, I think it might be a good idea to go ahead and have a mammogram."

"What's involved in that?" I asked.

"Well, you are standing during the test. The tech will place your breast on this plate, and then they have to push down on the top of your breast to flatten it out. It is a little bit uncomfortable, but it's necessary to do this so they can get a clear picture of the breast tissue."

"Sounds rather painful," I replied.

"Uncomfortable," he responded.

"Uncomfortable my ass," I thought as I chuckled to myself. "How would you know anyway?" I found his remark a bit ridiculous.

He handed me a piece of paper. "If you go to the front desk, they will give the order to you. We'll get back in contact with you once we receive the results. Should be within 2 or 3 days after it is done."

"OK, thanks," I said.

I took the order home and scheduled the test. The closer the date of the , the more anxious I became. My breast hurt just to touch them, and they are going to press down on them and flatten them out? That MUST be painful!

***

I hesitatingly entered the radiology office and gave my mammogram order to the lady behind the desk. My heart was racing, and I was a bit dizzy. She asked for my ID and insurance card, gave me some paperwork, and told me to fill it out. Since this occupied my mind, my anxiety waned for those few minutes. However, when all of the paperwork was filled out, the anxiety came back full force as I sat in the waiting room.

Finally, I was called back. The tech was quite friendly which again helped to ease my anxiety.

"OK, go into this room, take off your shirt and bra, and put on this robe. Make sure it opens in the front. You can put your belongings in this locker." She showed me how to lock it.

"OK," I said.

I slowly walked out of the room and looked down the hall.

"Ready?" she said. I turned around, and she was at the other end of the hall, walking in my direction.

"Yes," I responded.

She directed me into a room where this huge machine sat in the corner of the room. In front of it were two plastic-looking horizontal plates, one on top of the other with space in between the two.

"That must be where my breast is going," I thought to myself.

The tech went behind a plexiglass shield and typed something into a computer. I stood and waited for her, feeling even more dizzy. I could feel every heartbeat reverberate throughout my body.

She walked back into the room and directed me toward the machine.

"OK, we're going to start with the right breast. Open your robe and we're going to place your breast on top of this," she said, as she helped to place my breast on top of the bottom horizontal plate."

"Turn a little this way," she said as she adjusted the position of my breast. "OK, that's good."

Next, she pressed a button on the machine which brought the top plate down onto my breast. It started to become painful as I felt tremendous pressure on those sore lumps.

"You OK?" she asked.

"I'm OK," I responded. It hurt, but it was tolerable.

Next, she turned a knob on the side of the machine. This flattened my breast even more. I squished my face in pain, and the tech noticed it.

"I know this hurts, honey, but it will be over in just a few seconds. Bear with me."

"OK," I squeaked out.

"She quickly moved behind the plexiglass, told me to stop breathing, took the image, and returned to release the pressure on my breast.

"Thank God," I thought to myself.

"OK, now the left breast," she said. The same thing was done.

Once that was over, I thought, "Great. It's done." But I was wrong. She had to take two more images, this time from an angle. She moved the two horizontal plates until they were angled at about 60 degrees. These images, taken for each breast, were even more painful than the first two.

When the whole thing was over, I was so thankful. The severe anxiety subsided, but I was still worried about the results. Thankfully, those came rather quickly, and there was no cancer. It was just fibrocystic breast disease.

***

The attacks were becoming more frequent – every 2 to 3 months or so. The pain and bloating became much more severe. I fell into a depression and became so anxious during the end of my periods that I was almost afraid to leave my apartment. I was scared that an attack would happen when I wasn't close to a bathroom or out in public where I couldn't get home quickly. I also started to notice that red meat made me very nauseous during PMS. I assumed it was some kind of hormone fluctuation that caused this. If a steak was put in front of me during a bad bout of PMS, I usually would take only one bite and that was it. If I took another bite, I probably would have thrown up.

In addition to these symptoms, I noticed that during PMS, my allergy/sinus issues would worsen. I would sneeze more, become congested, and my nose would run. It was bad enough having all this abdominal pain and bloating, but to have that PLUS allergies/sinus congestion – well, I was purely miserable. I found myself in a brain fog during PMS. I was exhausted, unable to think clearly, and made mistakes at work that I wouldn't make during the other times of the month.

I returned to the gynecologist even though I knew I would have to have a Pap smear and pelvic exam if I did see him again. I was desperate. I had faith in doctors at that time, and I was sure this gynecologist would know exactly what was wrong and would be able to effectively treat me. I could not have been more wrong. This was just the very beginning of an exceptionally long, painful, highly educational, and life-changing journey.

The exam was painful, but this time, I did not hyperventilate. I knew what to expect. After his exam, the gynecologist explained in depth how prostaglandins can cause pain. After this lengthy explanation, he stated that NSAIDs block prostaglandins; therefore, NSAIDs should fix the problem. He prescribed Motrin®. I was despondent when I left. After that lengthy explanation that sounded so scientific, all he did was give me pain medication, something I had been using all along? You have got to be kidding me.

I went back to work, and my co-workers asked me what he said. I shared my story, and they all were in disbelief. We all talked about the ridiculousness of it. Little did I know that his reasoning for using Motrin were sound and correct. I realized this after years of research following my hysterectomy, but at the time, it just sounded like a pathetic attempt to get me out of his office.

> *Note:* **Prostaglandins are a type of lipid that is involved in the inflammatory process. They increase when there is tissue damage. An example is menstruation when endometrial tissue is broken down and released from the body during a period. These prostaglandins then cause the uterus to contract, causing pain in the form of menstrual cramps. Our body uses cyclooxygenase enzymes (COX) to produce prostaglandins from arachidonic acid. NSAIDS block COX enzymes which block the production of prostaglandins, thereby reducing pain.**

***

After several weeks, I returned to the gynecologist again and explained that the Motrin wasn't doing enough to combat the problem. He agreed to start me on birth control pills which he said should help to lessen the bleeding and hopefully help with the pain.

The first birth control pill did nothing but cause me to bleed for 2 weeks straight. I am unable to recall the name of this first birth control pill. I called the office.

"I've been bleeding for fifteen days straight, and I'm not slowing down. What do I do?" I asked the nurse.

"Well, sometimes it takes several months for your body to adjust to the pill. Give it a couple more months to see if your body will adjust to it."

I agreed to do this, but during the next several months, I stopped bleeding for about two weeks, bled for two weeks, and so forth. My cycle was a complete mess, and I was exhausted from all the blood loss. I returned once again to the gynecologist.

"I can't do this anymore. I am bleeding all the time, and I am exhausted. I've got to get this cycle straightened out."

I was switched to another birth control pill, and again, I am not able to recall the name of the pill.

"Give this one a couple of months. Hopefully, we'll have better luck this time," said the gynecologist.

I agreed once again to do this, but I was disheartened. During the next few months, I did have some irregular bleeding, but it was not as bad as the first pill that he had prescribed. However, I began to have frequent yeast infections which continued throughout my reproductive years.

***

I had become very frustrated with my gynecologist. My boyfriend's mother also had some menstrual issues, and she had been seeing a reproductive endocrinologist whose office was about an hour away from where I lived. She told me that this doctor had a great reputation and helped her, so I decided to schedule a visit with this reproductive endocrinologist.

On my drive to see the reproductive endocrinologist, my heart raced, and I felt nauseous. I knew I was going to have to endure another pelvic exam, and I knew it was going to hurt. Once I arrived at the office, I sat in the corner of the waiting room, crossed my legs, and shook the crossed leg constantly due to my anxiety. I was partly hunched over because of the nausea. I knew this was all stress-related, but I didn't know how to control it. I tried to breathe deeply which helped a little bit.

"You looked scared," said a teenage boy who sat next to his mother.

"What?" I asked.

"You looked scared. Are you OK?"

"Oh, I am fine," I said.

Did I actually look that bad? Was my anxiety so bad that a teenager could see it in my behavior? I stopped moving my leg and I adjusted myself in my seat. I didn't want the stress showing up in my behavior. I looked around at the other women. No one in the waiting room looked stressed at all. The women were all reading magazines, playing with their children, or nodding off. Why was this so stressful for me but not these other women? What was wrong with me that I couldn't endure a simple pelvic exam without pain and without severe anxiety? I felt so utterly alone.

I spent a long time with the reproductive endocrinologist as I explained the symptoms and concerns that I had for the past several years. She did a thorough exam and suggested that I once again change to a different birth control pill. She explained that each pill has differing amounts of estrogen and progesterone, and it would take some time to see which pill would work for me. She ordered some blood work and performed a pelvic exam which was painful. I thought this pain was part of being a woman, and to be honest, I was too embarrassed to ask if the pain was abnormal. That day, I went home with the birth control pill Orthocyclen®, and I waited for the results of the blood tests.

About a week later, the receptionist from the office called me. All of the blood work, including a CBC and thyroid test, came back normal. I was advised to stay on the current birth control pill for several months and allow my body to adjust to it.

***

I continued to bleed uncontrollably. Orthocyclen® wasn't helping much at all. After about four months, I returned to the reproductive endocrinologist.

Due to my excessive blood loss from taking different birth control pills, the reproductive endocrinologist decided to perform a D&C.

"Since your symptoms aren't improving, I think we should do a D&C," she said.

"Is that necessary?" I asked.

"Well, at this point, yes," she said. "I believe it is necessary to remove all the endometrium that has built up as a result of taking all of these different birth control pills," she said.

"What is involved in this?"

"We put you under general anesthesia, and I go in through the cervix and scrape the endometrial lining. This should dramatically decrease your bleeding after the surgery."

"Will I be in pain?"

"You may have some cramping after surgery, but we will have pain medication on hand, so it shouldn't be too bad."

"OK," I said with hesitation.

"Go to the front desk, and they will help you with all the necessary paperwork and will schedule the surgery, OK?"

"OK, I responded.

***

On my way to the hospital, thoughts raced through my head:

"How much pain will I be in when I wake up?"

"Will I ever be able to have children?"

"What if they have to remove my uterus?"

"What if they find cancer?"

In addition to being utterly terrified of having this surgery, I was also emotionally exhausted from all these "what ifs."

My heart raced as I waited to be taken back to surgery. I kept sighing deeply as that seemed to ease my anxiety a bit.

"What's wrong?" my mom asked.

"I'm just stressed. I can't wait for this to be over."

Finally, the time came. I was taken back to the operating room and put to sleep. When I woke up and was finally able to talk, I asked the nurses what the doctor found during the surgery.

"Just dysfunctional uterine bleeding. Nothing serious. You are going to be just fine."

It was a bittersweet moment for me. On one hand, nothing serious was found, but on the other hand, I still didn't know what was causing the pain. No one was able to give me a straight answer.

I remember having a lot of cramps after this surgery. I was given morphine and became extremely nauseated. I never vomited, but I came close. I also noticed that the pain relief I had lasted a very short time. I realized that it just wasn't worth it for me to take the morphine due to short-lived pain relief and extreme nausea. I would rather be in pain. I begged them to not give me any more morphine, and as my stomach settled down, I was given other pain medication which worked much better for me. The first time that I urinated, nothing but blood came out of me which again brought on the nausea. I almost passed out. This D&C did slow the bleeding, however, and for several years after this surgery.

> *Note*: **Many people have nausea after receiving morphine after surgery, so I am doubtful that this was an allergic reaction. However, as I was researching for this book, I found this study about morphine allergy and hormone levels, and I think it is a good idea to at least mention it here. Kalogeromitros et al. (1995) looked at 15 women with seasonal allergies and/or asthma who also had allergies to olive and parietaria (a plant from the nettle family that is also known as asthma weed because it has a high incidence of allergic reactions). The group compared them to 15 women without allergies (control group). They did skin prick tests with histamine and morphine. The skin pricks were done at three separate times in the menstrual cycle – during days 1-4, days 12-16, and days 24-28. There was a significant increase in weal and flare to histamine, morphine, and parietaria on days 12-16 which, interestingly, is the time of peak estrogen levels. This phenomenon occurred in all of the women, including controls.**

1992

"For adenomyosis, there's an... appalling lack of awareness and understanding of the disease, not just amongst the general public or women themselves, but also women's healthcare providers, ranging from GPs to imaging specialists, and even some gynecologists."

-Dr. Eisen Liang from his book, Could it be Adenomyosis? The (Bad) Cousin of Endometriosis

I met my husband in 1991, and we married in 1992. We lived in South Carolina until 1998. Although I had these menstrual issues, I never imagined that they would completely overtake my life. I just assumed at the time that eventually this would all be fixed once the doctors were able to figure out the problem.

Early in my marriage, I came home from work and fixed a spaghetti dinner. About 30 minutes after finishing the meal, my stomach bloated exactly the same way it had done in the past. Before I knew it, I was on the bathroom floor on all fours having severe contraction-like pain every two or three minutes. Sweat dripped off my face and onto the floor as I endured this horrible pain yet again. In between contractions, my husband opened the door and asked me if I was OK. As I sat on the floor, I told him no. I was in the middle of talking to him about what to do about this problem when another contraction hit.

"Another one's coming," I said as I got on my hands and knees. He stood there looking, and I told him to leave and close the door. After about an hour, I finally defecated, and the pain started to improve. I laid on the floor for about 15 minutes before I finally stood up and looked in the mirror. My hairline was soaked with sweat, my top was wet, and again, I was extremely pale.

I walked into the living room, and from the look on my husband's face, I could tell he was worried. I assured him I was fine now that the pain had stopped.

"Maybe it's something you ate?"

I shook my head in disgust.

"What if you drank more water?" he asked. "I mean, you complain of being constipated, so just drink more. Maybe take some Metamucil or something?"

"I have been using Metamucil," I responded.

I thought for a moment. What if I did drink more water? Maybe that would help.

I decided I would do that. I went to the store, bought a gallon plastic jug, and every day, I filled it with water. I took it to work, and every few hours, I would go into the employee kitchen, pull it out of the refrigerator, and I would drink as much as I could. My goal was to drink the entire gallon by the end of the day.

One day, I stood at the sink drinking my water, and my boss came in.

"Drinking all that water, huh?"

I swallowed. "Yep," I said. "I hope this will reduce my symptoms."

"I hope so too," she said.

Sadly, drinking more water did not help me. The attacks became increasingly frequent. They almost always occurred at the end of my period, so I was convinced that this was a gynecological issue. I knew symptoms were about to start when my stomach became extremely bloated. I knew that once the contractions started, the pain would not stop until I had a bowel movement which almost always ended with some degree of diarrhea.

1993

"...the now discredited mystery disorder presumed for centuries to be psychological in origin, was possibly endometriosis...this centuries-old notion linking chronic pelvic pain to mental illness exerted tremendous influence on attitudes about women with endometriosis in modern times, contributing to diagnostic delays and chronic indifference to their pain for most of the 20th century."

-Dr. Camran Nezhat

A few months later, I woke up again to searing abdominal pain. The pain was so severe that I prayed to God to get me through the cramps without passing out. Again, my shirt was soaked, and sweat was dripping off my face. My lower stomach was so bloated that anyone who saw me would have probably thought I was pregnant. This time, the nausea was so bad that I threw up several times during the attack. Finally, after a bout of diarrhea, the pain subsided, and I went back to bed. The next morning, I was exhausted. Later that day, I went to see the general practitioner once again.

"Something is seriously wrong. The pain is actually worse than what I remember when I had a ruptured appendix!"

"Well, this does sound like irritable bowel syndrome. I think you probably need to see a gastroenterologist."

"But it always happens during my period. Wouldn't that be a gynecological problem?"

"The symptoms sound exactly like IBS."

"Yes, but it always happens at the same time each month. And my uncle who did my appendectomy told me that if I ever had that kind of pain again, I should get medical help immediately."

"I understand, but it could just be a coincidence that it happens at the same time each month. Hormone fluctuations could also be setting off the IBS attacks. Let's just see what the gastroenterologist says."

As a scientist myself, this did make some sense to me; however, my gut told me that this diagnosis wasn't correct. Call it instinct or whatever – he just didn't quite get it in my opinion. I was so annoyed! Here I was, having severe abdominal pain that was worse than what I had with my ruptured appendix, and no one could give me a definitive diagnosis. I took a deep breath and tried to calm myself down. Maybe the problem was in the gastrointestinal tract. I had to remind myself that I needed to look at any possibility. I left that day with a referral, and I went home and made the appointment.

I shared my reservations about the diagnosis with my husband, but I didn't think he really understood either. I felt so lost and alone. Little did I know that these feelings would eventually become so powerful as to completely rule my life.

***

One night, my husband and I went to my in-laws' house for dinner. After dinner, we sat in their family room and talked.

"Well, it looks like I am going to have a colonoscopy."

"Oh, you don't want that," said my mother-in-law. "You better run the other direction if they want to do that to you!"

"What? Why?" I asked. I was already scared of this procedure, and my mother-in-law quickly increased my dread.

"Oh, I had that done years ago," she said. I was on my knees…on all fours…and they put that tube up my behind. It was awful! It was extremely painful!"

"Are you serious?" I asked.

"Dead serious."

"Is it done that way now?" I asked as I looked at my husband. He shrugged his shoulders.

"I don't know," said my mother-in-law. "All I know is you better run the opposite direction if they try to do that to you!"

I left their house that night feeling like I was on the verge of a nervous breakdown. I had all this pain, and the only way they may be able to help me is with a colonoscopy. I was petrified.

***

PMS was getting worse. I was extremely moody during the week before menstruation, and stress at work along with the pain and heavy bleeding was just making it worse. Sinus issues were driving me insane. It is awful to be in pain, feeling like you want to cry, and sniffing every five seconds because your nose is running nonstop. One day, my husband suggested I consider starting an antidepressant.

"Why don't you just try it?" he asked. "It might make you feel so much better."

I was young, and I did consider it. After all, some of my other co-workers were on anti-depressants, and they seem to feel better on them. At the time, it was kind of the "thing to do." Eventually, I agreed to this, thinking that it might help me to deal with all the stress I was under at that time.

I went to my general practitioner and discussed the use of antidepressants for my depression. He agreed that this type of medication may help me, so he put me on Paxil®. I did see a slight reduction in my mood swings, but as time went on, the mood swings became worse. Eventually, he switched me to Zoloft® which seemed to work better for me.

1994

"Many patients have seen gastroenterologists...for assessment of possible GI causes of their pain, often more than one doctor, having extensive testing including CT scans, endoscopies, colonoscopies, GI motility studies, MRI enterography, etc., often costing thousands of dollars. If the initial doctor would focus on the underlying pelvic pain, they would understand that endometriosis is often the most common diagnosis."

-Dr. Ken Sinervo

The gastroenterologist was very personable and seem genuinely concerned about me and all the pain that I had endured. He agreed that I needed a colonoscopy to see if there was any abnormality in the large intestine. He was also particularly concerned about residual problems from my ruptured appendix. He talked to me about the possibility of an intestinal obstruction as a result of the ruptured appendix – just as I had thought on the night of my first attack. I absolutely dreaded the thought of having this procedure done, but when you are in such pain, believe me, you will agree to do just about any medical procedure to find a solution.

A few weeks later, I began the prep for the colonoscopy. This involved drinking an exceptionally large container of medicated liquid which caused me to have constant bowel movements most of the night. This was the worst part of the test. I had to drink 8 ounces of this liquid every twenty minutes until it was gone. About halfway through the container, I became very cold and walked around the house with a big blanket wrapped around me. I started to have bowel movements ever 15 minutes or so which quickly turned to repeated bouts of diarrhea. When I got close to the bottom of the container, I was so nauseated that I couldn't finish it. At that point, nothing was coming out of my gastrointestinal tract except water. I had thoroughly cleaned myself out, so not finishing the container had no negative impact on the actual colonoscopy.

The next morning, I was both nauseated and extremely anxious. I couldn't wait until this test was over. The gastroenterologist put me into a light sleep, and I didn't remember most of the procedure. There was a fleeting moment where I was jerked awake for a second, and I remember feeling a little bit of pain in the upper part of my abdomen, but I quickly fell back to sleep. When I woke up, I felt fine – no nausea and no pain. After the procedure, he told us that I had a healthy colon. He also told my husband and I that the appendix area was fine without any adhesions present. He could find no abnormality at all in the colon that would explain my episodes of pain. Although this should have been good news, I felt bothered because I still did not have a reason for my episodes of severe abdominal pain.

When the gastroenterologist gave me the results, he noticed the disappointed look on my face.

"This is good news, Maria," he said. "You should be happy."

"I still don't have an answer to what is causing my pain," I replied.

He explained that at least I know that it isn't something serious in the gastrointestinal tract. That gave little comfort to me, a person who was dealing with excruciating pain, nausea, constipation, diarrhea, and sometimes vomiting on almost a monthly basis at that point. He gave me the antispasmodic drug Levsin® to take during the attacks of pain. His opinion was that I may have been suffering from irritable bowel syndrome – just as my general practitioner has suspected.

> ***Medication facts:*** **Levsin®, also known as hyoscyamine, is an anticholinergic drug used to treat gastrointestinal disorders including irritable bowel syndrome. Specifically, it inhibits the action of acetylcholine on smooth muscles.**

Note: According to Dr. Ken Sinervo with the Center for Endometriosis Care, about 5 to 10% of invasive endometriosis cases may involve the appendix. Dr. Sinervo also states that a colonoscopy is rarely helpful when diagnosing endometriosis. Milone et al. (2015) states that only 4% of invasive bowel lesions are detected using this procedure. In addition, Dr. Tamer Seckin (2020) states, "...endoscopy really looks inside the bowel and doesn't see the outside of the bowel, which we see in our laparoscopy, we see all these lesions. Even though they are on the bowel or retroperitoneum, there is no way this colonoscopist or GI doctor will diagnose endometriosis." Dr. Camran Nezhat (2021) confirms this view. He states, "Colonoscopies have particularly high fail rates in detecting bowel endometriosis, since most of the growths occur on the outside of the bowel, rather than inside it."

***

After the colonoscopy, I noticed a clear change in my co-workers. I specifically remember a time when I walked into the lab, and I noticed three of them talking quietly. When they saw me, they all became quiet and then walked away from each other. I knew they were talking about me, but I ignored them. I just kept the hurt bottled up inside me. I later found out that a group of them had been gossiping about me, saying that I was "faking it". Since the doctors could not find the cause of my pain, they assumed I was making it all up.

A couple of my friends had talked to me about endometriosis around this time because another friend had been diagnosed with it, and my symptoms sounded similar to her symptoms. They had heard that pregnancy may improve symptoms, so they suggested that I try and get pregnant. This idea intrigued me, so I talked to my husband about it, and we decided to try for pregnancy. I came off the Orthocyclen®, and the bleeding became worse – I would bleed for about 12 days each month, and 3 of those days would be extremely heavy. I would also have spotting for several days between each period. I continued to have attacks of debilitating pain toward the end of my period. Some months, the pain was extremely severe, and other months, the pain was moderate. I did my best to keep my chin up as I was hopeful that pregnancy would help my symptoms.

1995

"Behind every chronic illness is just a person trying to find their way in the world. We want to find love and be loved and be happy just like you. We want to be successful and do something that matters. We're just dealing with unwanted limitations in our hero's journey."

-Glenn Schweitzer

Our friends and/or family members had the habit of just dropping by to visit. They would not call ahead. It didn't matter that we were in the middle of dinner. It didn't matter if we had a particularly difficult day at work. It didn't matter if I was in the middle of a horrible period. We were expected to just stop whatever we were doing and to entertain. Sometimes these friends and family members stayed for hours. It wasn't uncommon for some of them to stay until 11 p.m. or so when we had to get up early for work the next day. One time, when I was on my period, I just told them that I had to go to bed. I stood up and politely excused myself, saying they were welcome to stay and talk to my husband, which is what they did. I just couldn't stay up any longer. I literally couldn't hold my eyes open. My husband seemed a little agitated, but I didn't care anymore. The next day at work was agonizing. I was completely exhausted and found myself making stupid mistakes because I could not concentrate from the lack of sleep and excessive blood loss. I think back on it now, and I honestly do not know how I did it.

***

I pulled the sheets back and left the bedroom doubled over as to not disturb my husband. I crawled up the stairs to our guest bedroom, and just as I lay down, another cramp hit. I writhed in pain as I waited for the severe cramp to pass. I knew I was going to be in excruciating pain for hours, and there was no way to stop it.

I lay down on my right side, but it felt like that was aggravating the cramping pain, so I turned to my left side. I had a brief few minutes of pain relief, but the nausea was unrelenting. Suddenly, I felt that horrendous cramping pain begin. I lay there in the fetal position, and I was seriously hoping for death. Death would be better than this. I tried to roll over again, hoping that would help relieve the pain, but it made it worse. I got out of bed and walked, doubled over, while clutching my lower abdomen. I grabbed the wall, then the sink, and I was able to sit down on the toilet before I almost passed out. By that time, the cramp had passed. I sat on the toilet, sweat pouring down the sides of my face, and I tried to push. The urge to defecate was overwhelming. I pushed and pushed, but nothing happened. I put my face in my hands and began to cry.

Another cramp hit me. I doubled over while I sat on the toilet. I felt like my intestines were going to rupture. This was the worst pain yet.

Since I was unable to defecate, I slowly made my way back to the guest bedroom. I sat down on the small couch and curled up into a ball. When was this agony going to stop? I rocked back and forth. I don't know why I did this, but in some weird way, it gave me a little bit of comfort.

Another cramp. This time the nausea overtook me, and I quickly returned to the bathroom where I threw up. I cleaned myself up in between the severe cramps.

I was exhausted, but the cramping continued. A few minutes of relief, and then bam – another cramp. They started on my left side, and some would continue into my lower back or down into the left side of my pelvis. I sat on the toilet and pushed to no avail, so then I would walk around, doubled over, thinking that this might help. When I couldn't walk anymore, I would lay down, and this would go on for hours and hours.

"If only I could defecate," I thought. "Then the pain would stop."

I returned to the bathroom and pushed as hard as I could, but nothing came out. Another cramp. I stopped pushing and just tried to breathe through the cramp and nausea. As the cramp let up, I pushed and pushed again. Another cramp. I was doubled over on the toilet as sweat dripped down my face and onto the floor. My shirt was soaked with sweat. As the cramp let up, I pushed as hard as I could. Finally, I was able to defecate.

"Thank God," I said to myself. Exhausted, I returned to the guest bedroom and lay down, hoping that defecation would help reduce the pain.

A few minutes later, a huge cramp took over my lower abdomen, and I felt the urgent need to defecate. I quickly returned to the bathroom and had a huge bout of diarrhea.

"What the hell?" I said to myself. "One minute I am horribly constipated, and the next I am having diarrhea! What the hell is wrong with me?"

After this, I returned to the bedroom, and the cramps quickly subsided. I fell asleep. The next morning, I felt as if I had run a marathon. There was no way I could work after going through that.

***

About a month later, I took the first of many pregnancy tests. Sadly, it was negative. We were disappointed, but we had also been told that it was common for it to take several months to get pregnant. We knew we would have to try for up to a year before going on fertility drugs. So, we just kept trying.

About the 4th month of trying, we decided to increase our odds. After intercourse, I laid on the bed upside down with my legs resting on the headboard. We laughed as we "encouraged" the egg and sperm to come together.

Even after our extra efforts, the pregnancy tests continued to come back negative. It finally got to the point that I expected a negative test, and I started to really wonder if we would be able to have children.

> *Note*: **Infertility is defined as a failure to achieve a pregnancy after 12 months of unprotected sexual intercourse.**

My fibrocystic disease was getting worse and worse. Some months it was so bad that I didn't want my husband to even hug me. Even though I told him about my sore breasts, he either didn't listen or didn't care because he always forgot about it.

"Careful!" I exclaimed as my husband embraced me.

"What?" he said.

"My breasts," I would say, irked as this had been probably the 10th time I told him about this problem.

"Oh," he said as he loosened his embrace.

This would happen repeatedly, and my frustration with him grew to almost intolerable levels each time I had to remind him to be careful. I kept my irritation bottled up inside. I felt alone and completely invisible. Who in my life really "saw" the true me? Who really "saw" the person with this health problem?

Sex was something I started to dread each month during PMS. It just wasn't enjoyable at all for me. Intercourse during that time felt like a hot, burning pain. I also had tearing sensations in the back part of my vagina. When I urinated after having sex, I felt burning and stinging pain which hurt so bad that I dreaded going to the bathroom. I wanted my husband to be happy, though, so I would just put up with the pain. To this day, I know he didn't have even an inkling of the pain I had to endure during and after intercourse.

***

Some of my other co-workers were getting pregnant, and I envied them. When would that day come for me? We continued to try, and then one month, I was convinced that I was pregnant. Even though I suffered from heavy bleeding and pain, I was very regular – every twenty-eight to thirty days. Most of the time it was 28 days on the nose. However, one month, I was late. I took a pregnancy test, and it was negative. Then there was no period on day 32, then day 33, then day 34.

"I have to be pregnant," I told my husband. "I am now on day 34, and no bleeding!"

We tried not to get too excited because my pregnancy tests were all negative before this. But I was never this late, and I felt exhausted. Also, my breasts were hurting particularly bad, and a couple of my friends told me that was a sign of pregnancy. Could this be the month?

On the morning of day 35, I woke up to spotting. I was devastated. I had really convinced myself that I was pregnant. My period was particularly heavy and prolonged that month, and to this day, I wondered if I was pregnant but had an early miscarriage.

***

After repeated trips to the reproductive endocrinologist, I became despondent, miffed, and extremely moody. It just seemed as if there were no answers. My co-worker's attitudes toward me just fed into my anxiety and depression. It was an awful time.

One night, as my mother-in-law and I sat in my car while we waited outside her friend's house (we waited for her to get home because she was going to cut our hair), I decided to open up to her about what I was going through. I explained to her how bad the pain had become. I told her about the extremely heavy bleeding, about how perplexed I was that I did not know what was causing these symptoms, and about how depression was setting in. I explained that our attempts to become pregnant have failed so far. I told her about how my co-workers had been acting toward me and how they thought that since the doctors could not find the cause, I must be "faking it." I was deeply hurt and even more depressed when she responded, "Well, I just think that you should have kids. Just get pregnant. The two of you would make such great parents. You just need to have kids." I knew at that point that my mother-in-law didn't understand it either. I knew that all she wanted was grandchildren, and it seemed like it didn't matter to her what I was going through. In addition, she had no clue what was happening privately between my husband and I with all these negative pregnancy tests. She had no idea how hurtful her comments were that night. If she had only listened, she would have had a better understanding of how hard we were trying to have children. It was at that point that I decided not to share any other details of my condition with her or really anyone. It was like I built a giant wall around me. I was slowly blocking people from insight into my health issue because I was afraid of being hurt and rejected. I started to push all my emotions deep down inside me.

> ***What we know today*: It is now known that endometriosis is one of the top causes of female infertility. Adenomyosis is also known to play a role**

in infertility. This topic is discussed at length later in this book.

***Note*: In a study by Moradi et al. (2014), endometriosis patients stated that "Their family and friends also told them that pain and bleeding were normal, and their doctors misdiagnosed or mistreated them because they normalized symptoms and did not believe them, or they lacked knowledge."**

***

My parents traveled from Wisconsin to South Carolina to visit us for Christmas that year. My sister also came along with my brother and his wife. I was so excited to host Christmas at my house.

I wanted to make sure that my period would not interfere with my Christmas plans, so I took Advil and Midol every day as a preventative. We all had a wonderful time the first day. However, I had another attack on the second day. I woke up in the middle of the night in severe pain again. I could not believe it! Even after taking Advil and Midol consistently, I STILL had an attack. I was so angered and depressed. Once again, I was exhausted the next day, so I had to take a nap. When I woke up, I heard everyone in the kitchen. They were laughing and really enjoying themselves while I laid in bed, exhausted from the nightmare that I had endured the night before. Sadness enveloped me as I realized how this health issue had impacted my quality of life.

I finally got up and joined the fun. I had not showered and was in my pajamas, so I felt ugly and dirty, but my mom insisted that I join them regardless. We ended up playing a game that night which was quite enjoyable, but I still could not manage to get out of my funk. I was just so sick and tired of dealing with this beast inside me.

1996

*"When IBS is symptomatic and flares up during periods,
endometriosis should be considered seriously."*

-Dr. Tamer Seckin

In 1996, the attacks occurred on pretty much a monthly basis. It was the toughest part of my journey. I missed work quite a bit which just added to the negative attitude that my co-workers had toward me. I dreaded going in to work and having to face them each day. I was hurting, heartbroken, and lonely.

***

My husband and I went to my in-laws one night to celebrate my mother-in-law's birthday. I remember not feeling quite right, but I still felt well enough to attend. About 30 minutes after dinner, I suddenly became very nauseated. I started to feel those dreaded symptoms – the bloating, the pain, the nausea – and I knew we had to get home immediately. I told my husband that we had to leave, and I remember the whole family seemed to be a little bothered, especially my husband. We made it home in time for me to run upstairs and vomit.

I think my husband's tolerance for this illness had grown short at this point. In between the waves of pain, I walked out of the bathroom an into the adjacent guest bedroom where my husband was surfing the internet. I told him that I had just vomited.

"Really?" he said without taking his eyes off the computer screen.

"Yes," I responded. "It's happening again."

"Can I do anything?" he responded, again without taking his eyes off the computer screen.

Disturbed, I answered, "No." I returned to the bathroom where I remained for the next several hours – vomiting, in pain, sweating, culminating in a horrible case of diarrhea. When it was finally over, I walked out of the bathroom and into the guest bedroom where I crawled into bed. My husband had already turned off the computer and gone to bed in the master bedroom. He never checked on me.

Interestingly, several weeks later, I saw some pictures taken at the party, and I noticed that my stomach looked very bloated. I looked like I was about 3 to 4 months pregnant. The picture had been taken about 15 minutes before dinner. I was so embarrassed.

***

Eventually, the reproductive endocrinologist agreed to perform a laparoscopy to see if she could determine the cause of my pain. She explained that during the surgery, she would look around the outside area of the appendix and see if there were any adhesions that may be causing some of the pain.

> ***What we know today:*** **We now know that endometriosis, because of constant inflammation in the peritoneum, can lead to adhesions. The topic of adhesions will be discussed further later in this book.**

Once again, I was scared. The same questions kept me awake at night, playing repeatedly in my head:

"What if they find something serious like cancer?"

"What if I can't have children?"

"When am I going to get an answer, and when is this all going to be over?"

"Will I ever have a normal life?"

"Will I be in pain when I wake up?"

"Will I be nauseated when I wake up?"

It was like a record – the same thoughts playing over and over in my mind. These thoughts only intensified the extreme stress I was already under at that time.

I remember waking up in recovery, and I shook uncontrollably. This had not happened during the D&C, so I was confused.

"She's been doing that since she came out of surgery," a nurse said. My eyes were closed, but I could hear them talk.

"Wow, that's unusual," said another nurse.

What was wrong with me? Why was I so cold? I felt someone put a warm, heavy blanket on me which felt so good. I opened my eyes.

"Maria?" asked the nurse.

"Yeah," I responded in a whisper.

"You're in recovery. You did great."

"What did they find?" I asked, barely able to get the words out.

"Um, hold on," she responded. "Let me look in the chart."

She walked away, and I dozed off. I noticed that my shaking wasn't nearly as bad since that heavy blanket had been placed on top of me.

"Maria?" said the nurse.

I woke back up and slowly opened my eyes.

"Looks like you have polycystic ovarian syndrome."

"Oh," I responded, not knowing what that was.

"Your doctor will come in and talk to you about it soon," she said.

"OK," I said as I closed my eyes and drifted back off to sleep.

The next time I woke up, I heard my mother-in-law speaking to my husband.

"She better get that blood pressure up," she said. "92 over 55?"

I dozed back off to sleep.

"They aren't going to let her go home with that blood pressure down like that." She was still commenting on it when I woke up a second time.

I didn't react to her comments and actually was a bit amused by it. I have always had low blood pressure. My normal pressure at the time was about 90/60, but she didn't know that. She was panicking over nothing.

"Maria?" asked the nurse.

I opened my eyes.

"Do you know what your normal blood pressure is?"

"About 90 over 60 usually," I whispered.

"She's fine," said the nurse. My mother-in-law never made another comment.

As I started to fully wake up, I heard another patient across from me moan as she woke up from surgery. Suddenly, I heard her vomit and a nurse yelled, "I need suction!"

"Oh, that's awful," said my mother-in-law.

My husband closed the curtain so we wouldn't have to see or hopefully hear anything else.

"Why is she vomiting? We aren't supposed to eat past midnight before surgery," I said.

"Maybe she didn't do what she was supposed to do," said my mother-in-law.

"Maybe," I said. "Or some people just can't handle anesthesia."

I realized how lucky I was at that time. I woke up with no nausea, and I was hungry.

About thirty minutes later, a nurse came in and asked how I was feeling.

"Pretty good so far," I said.

"Do you want to try a few crackers and a sprite?"

"Sure," I responded. "By the way, what is polycystic ovarian syndrome?"

"Um," said the nurse. My husband and mother-in-law looked at me with confusion on their faces.

"The nurse in recovery said I had polycystic ovarian syndrome."

"Um, the doctor needs to talk to you about that," said the nurse.

I ate the crackers and drank the sprite, and I had no issues. I was really shocked that I did not have any nausea or much pain; however, I was on pain meds, so I wondered how much pain I would be in after the meds wore off.

The doctor finally came in to talk to me.

"Well, you had a little bit of endometriosis," she said. "That is what is probably causing your symptoms."

"Just a little bit?" I asked, confused. How could just a little bit of endometriosis cause such severe pain?

"Yes, just a little on your ovary and on your uterus. The amount of pain has nothing to do with how much endometriosis is present. Some women have just a little bit and have severe pain, and other women have it all over and have very little pain."

"Really? That's strange," I said.

"We don't know why that is, but that's what happens."

"What about polycystic ovarian syndrome?" I asked.

My doctor looked at me, puzzled.

"The recovery room nurse said I had polycystic ovarian syndrome."

"No, that's not right," she responded. "No, all you have is endometriosis."

"Oh, OK," I responded.

"Sure you didn't dream that?" asked my husband.

"No, I swear that's what she said!"

"She may have had the wrong chart," said my doctor. "We ablated those endometrial implants, so you should be feeling much better very soon."

"That's great," I responded, feeling relieved.

About an hour later, the nurse returned and asked if I wanted to try and go to the bathroom. I agreed, and I expected to have no issues since I had come out of this surgery without any real problems except for feeling cold when I woke up.

She wheeled my stretcher right next to the bathroom door, and she helped me to sit up on the side of the bed.

"Do you feel dizzy?" she asked.

"No, I think I am OK," I responded.

"Take it slowly," she responded.

I sat there for about 30 seconds, and then she helped me to stand up.

"Do you still feel OK?" she asked.

"Yeah, I am fine," I responded.

"OK, I will be right here when you are finished," she said.

I walked into the bathroom, rolling the IV bag holder alongside of me. I sat down on the toilet and urinated without much of a problem. However, when I stood back up, I suddenly became dizzy and a little nauseated. I opened the door and told the nurse.

"OK, that's normal," she said as she helped me to get back up on the stretcher. "Just lay back."

As I lied back on the stretcher, I felt so nauseated. Luckily, the nausea did not last. It resolved quickly, but this caused anxiety in me. I was afraid it would happen again when I stood up to go home.

I continued to rest for about another hour and then was released to go home. Even though I was nervous about standing again, the dizziness and nausea never returned.

During the operation, my surgeon performed a tubal insufflation to make sure the fallopian tubes were open. She did this because we had been trying for a pregnancy and had not had any luck. The good news was that the tubes were found to be open without any kind of blockage that might be contributing to my infertility.

> *Note:* **A tubal insufflation, also known as Rubin's test, refers to the inflation of the fallopian tubes with carbon dioxide gas to make sure the tubes are fully open and not blocked.**

> *What is known today:* **Endometriosis is a condition where endometrial-like cells found are found outside of the uterus. Common sites of implants are the ovaries, bladder, bowel, rectum, and the outside of the uterus. This procedure was done in 1996 at a time when excision of endometriosis was not routinely done. At that time, if any endometriosis was found,**

an ablation was done. The difference between an ablation and excision was explained to me in a great way – an ablation is when you "cut the grass." An excision is when you "pull up the grass by its roots." So, if you ablate endometriosis implants, they will eventually grow back. If you excise them, they will not grow back if all implants are excised. Excision is the gold standard treatment of endometriosis today.

***

My husband had to work during my recovery, so my mother-in-law came over and sat with me during the day. Because I was on pain medication, I wanted to sleep most of the time, so that's what I did. When I woke up around lunch time, my mother-in-law asked if I wanted something to eat.

"Yes, that would be great," I responded.

She went to the kitchen and came back a few minutes later with a tray that had a sandwich and chips on it. I pulled myself up to a sitting position and immediately noticed pain in my shoulders.

"Are you OK?" she asked. She had noticed a grimace on my face.

"Yeah, my shoulders just hurt," I responded as I massaged them. "Must have been how I was lying."

The pain felt like a deep ache. It reminded me of the type of achy pain that I felt the day after I had a particularly hard dance class or aerobics class.

She placed the food in my lap, and I ate all of it, but I continued to notice the achy pain in my shoulders.

"It's weird," I said. "It feels like I've been to the gym and worked my shoulders out like crazy."

"That's strange," she said.

"I know."

After lunch, I lay back down on the couch and noticed that the shoulder pain was better.

"It's better now."

"Good," she responded. "Do you need anything else?"

"No, I am fine."

> ***Note***: **During a laparoscopy, CO2 gas is injected into the abdomen so that the surgeon can visualize the abdominal organs during the surgery. Some gas may remain in the body for several days, and it can cause pain post-surgery. The pain is normally better when lying down, and it increases when sitting up because the gas rises. Therefore, pain is often felt in the shoulders. The gas dissipates over the course of several days, and the pain resolves usually with minimal to no treatment.**

"Any channel you want to watch?"

"No, I am probably going back to sleep."

"Just sleep as much as you need to," she responded.

I wanted to sleep for two reasons. First, I was loopy from the pain medication. Second, I didn't want to get into any in-depth discussion about children. I knew she would push the matter again, and it really upset me. I felt like a loser that I couldn't give a child to my husband, and I sure didn't want to hear someone go on and on about how we should have children. At the time, I thought we would be great parents. But I was having a very real internal struggle. I had to face the fact that we may never be able to have children.

***

During my follow-up appointment after the laparoscopy, the reproductive endocrinologist reiterated that she did find some endometriosis on the ovaries and uterus. She explained again that the degree of endometriosis does not determine the degree of pain. She showed me pictures that she took during the surgery and said that other than the few endometriosis implants, the uterus and ovaries appeared normal. Her opinion was that the source of the pain was endometriosis.

I had little pain for the next two months, and I was optimistic that this surgery would be the end of this nightmare. Sadly, three months after surgery, the severe pain came back full force.

I woke up to the contraction pain once again. I quietly got up, went upstairs to the guest bedroom, and began the horrendous three-to-four-hour journey to hell and back. This was one of my worst attacks. At one point, the pain was so bad that I thought my intestines were certainly going to rupture. That is the one contraction that is still vivid in my mind today. It was on my right side, and I held onto the door of the guest bedroom, shaking, and feeling incredibly faint at the height of it. The pain was indescribable. I really thought that was the one that would finally kill me, but right when I thought that, the contraction lessened. My heart raced, and I started to cry. If a contraction like that happened again, surely something in there would rupture. I was convinced of that.

I was vomiting, pushing extremely hard in between contractions to try to defecate, and almost fainted two or three times. I knew I needed to go to the hospital, but I knew I would never make it down the stairs to wake up my husband. Then I heard some noise – he had gotten up to use the bathroom!

"Thank God," I thought as sweat dripped down my face. I hoped that after he used the bathroom, he would come and check on me.

But he didn't. Instead, he just went back to bed, and I didn't have the energy to walk downstairs to get him.

I ended up getting through it, but I realized that night that I was on my own. His lack of compassion just made it that much more difficult to deal with the pain. I needed empathy. I desperately needed someone who listened and genuinely cared.

***

The gossip continued in the lab. It became so bad that when I asked for help in processing specimens, almost no one would help me except for a select few. I remember asking my husband what he thought since he used to work at the same place. He ended up telling me that one of my co-workers who had cancer and beat it was speaking badly about me. She compared my situation to her situation, saying that if she was able to beat cancer, then I should just suck it up and keep going. She had absolutely no idea the amount of pain I had to endure!

It became unbearable. Not only was I faced with extremely heavy bleeding and unrelenting severe pain for which I did not know the cause, but I was also going into a hostile work environment and was dealing with a husband who lacked compassion all while trying desperately hold my head up and act like everything was alright. It wasn't. It was far from alright. Many nights, I cried quietly in bed. I wanted so badly to run away. Many times, I thought about doing it. But the reality was that no matter how far I ran, whatever this thing was that was inside of me will always be there. I would never be able to run away from this relentless pain, this limitless bleeding, this hideous monster inside me.

> **Note: According to Sinaii et al (2002), 22% of women in the general population are unable to work during menstruation. However, "By comparison, 81% of [endometriosis] survey respondents were unable to work, including doing household chores, because of**

***

I returned to the reproductive endocrinologist for another exam. I explained that my symptoms were the same. As usual, the Pap smear and pelvic exam were quite painful. It was virtually impossible for me to relax during these exams. After the Pap smear, she inserted her finger into my vagina and asked me if it hurt. She pressed on the back of my vagina, and I almost came off the table. It hurt so bad! She said, "OK", removed her finger and told me to get dressed. She did not address why it pained me so much when she pressed on the back of my vagina. I always wondered why she did that. What was she thinking, and why didn't she follow up on it?

> *Note*: **I learned later about endometriosis that is present in the rectovaginal pouch. Rectovaginal endometriosis is endometriosis in the cul-de-sac or the area between the back of the vagina and the bowel.**
>
> **When the reproductive endocrinologist pressed on the back of my vagina, why didn't that alert her to the possible presence of rectovaginal endometriosis? Did she notice this symptom and then forget to address it? I wish I knew the answer, and I really regret why she asked me that question.**
>
> **This may have been a clear missed opportunity to really investigate and discover what was going on with me. Rectovaginal endometriosis is discussed further later in this book.**

***

While dealing with all the intense pain and heavy bleeding, I also dealt with oppressive and continual exhaustion. There were times when I worked exceptionally long days in the lab, and when I arrived home, I would try to sneak in a nap before my husband came home. These small naps didn't help much though. When I woke up, I still felt totally drained. At times when watching movies at night, I could barely hold my eyes open, and I would end up falling asleep. My husband made comments to me about how he was irked that I would sleep during movies, but he never understood how utterly drained I was from the pain and the massive blood loss. This put extra pressure on me to keep my husband happy which made this whole situation that much more burdensome. I fought extremely hard to stay awake during movies and/or TV shows to make him feel wanted and special. But the thing I realize today, after many years of counseling, is that my needs were not being met.

One night, I had an unusual attack which only happened once in those dreadful 17 years. I woke up in the middle of the night once again, bloated and in pain, but I was also extraordinarily dizzy. I slowly crawled up the stairs to the guest bedroom. I had to stop several times and put my head between my legs because I was so close to fainting. Once I made it to the bedroom, I sat in the computer chair with my head between my legs. The pain wasn't quite as bad as it had been, but the dizziness was debilitating. After about 5 minutes of sitting with my head between my legs, I sat up and immediately felt like I was going to faint. I quickly put my head between my legs again and just sat there, afraid to sit up. After about 30 minutes or so, I slowly lifted my head and stood up, doubled over. I walked over to the bed and lay down. I started to feel faint again, so I hung my head off the side of the bed. I was still bloated, but the pain was bearable, so I closed my eyes. I eventually drifted off to sleep, and when I woke up, my head was still hanging off the side of the bed. I decided to move my head to the pillow, and I didn't feel faint. I fell asleep. The attack was over.

Note: I am not sure what exactly happened during this attack. Could it have been anemia? Maybe. After

all, the attack occurred at the end of my period, and I always had extremely heavy periods. Was it a vasovagal reaction? Maybe. I am just not sure what triggered this kind of reaction.

***

I returned to my general practitioner and explained that these attacks were having a terrible impact on my mental health. I had begun to have what I now believe are panic attacks. If I was out in public and my stomach became bloated or my abdomen started to hurt, I started to feel panicky. My heart would start to race, and I would get shaky and dizzy. I would also become nauseated. As soon as the first little symptom reared its ugly head, no matter where I was, I immediately went home if I could. I was petrified of an imminent attack.

During this visit, the general practitioner confirmed the diagnosis of irritable bowel syndrome. He refilled my prescription for the antispasmodic drug Levsin® to take when an attack started.

"This should really help with the pain that you are feeling during these attacks. It helps to calm the muscles in the GI tract and prevents them from going into spasm," said the general practitioner as he handed me the prescription.

I had taken Levsin® once since my colonoscopy, but it didn't do much to reduce my symptoms. I didn't have much hope for this drug, but I was willing to give it another try.

Levsin® did not work at all the second time I took it. It did nothing to stop the pain, so I went back to the general practitioner. This time he gave me a prescription for Bentyl®. I had absolutely no knowledge of these medications, and I trusted my doctors. However, as I learned later, Bentyl® was also an antispasmodic just like Levsin.

> ***Medication facts:*** **Bentyl®, also known as dicyclomine, is an anticholinergic drug used in the**

treatment of irritable bowel syndrome. It causes the smooth muscle in the gastrointestinal tract to relax by blocking a chemical present in the intestines.

***

Since I was having so many health issues, my husband suggested that we take a vacation to Las Vegas to help reduce my stress level. I was nervous about traveling, but I agreed to go for the simple fact that I just wanted to get away from work for a while. Maybe this is what I needed – a reprieve from stress. My in-laws decided to meet us there.

The vacation was a lot of fun, and luckily, I didn't have any issues until we were getting ready to fly home. I woke up that morning feeling a little bloated. I felt like that time when we went to my mother-in-law's birthday party.

"Oh, please cooperate with me," I silently said to my body. "At least until we get home!"

At breakfast, I made sure I ate healthy food – lots of fruit, especially fruits like pineapple which have a lot of fiber. I drank a ton of water. I did anything I could think of to make sure I didn't have another attack. After breakfast, I went back to the room and tried my hardest to have a bowel movement.

"If I could just have a bowel movement," I thought, "I think I'd be OK until I got home."

I had no such luck. I pushed and pushed, but there was nothing. I started to panic a little, but I did some deep breathing exercises and was able to calm myself down.

We made it to the airport. I still felt "off", so I tried once again to have a bowel movement at the airport. Again, nothing happened. Nausea started to kick in, and I started to shake. I returned to the check-in line and told my husband that I didn't think I would be able to fly.

"What? We're already here. Just get on the plane, and you can sleep all the way home."

"No, I can't do this," I replied. "I'm too nauseous."

"Let's go sit down," replied my mother-in-law. "You'll be fine if we just sit down for a minute."

"No, really. I know how this goes. I'm going to be in a lot of pain soon!"

"We'll go get her a soda. That will help," replied my mother-in-law.

I glared at my husband. "Listen to me! I CAN'T FLY! I AM SICK!"

My husband reluctantly left the line with me.

"You all go on," he said to his parents. "We'll get another flight."

He took me back to the hotel and explained the situation to the person at the front desk. While he did that, I went back to the bathroom and desperately tried to have a bowel movement. I pushed extremely hard, but nothing happened yet again. I was so agitated, but I knew if I didn't calm down, it would just get worse. I continued with the deep breathing exercises.

We were able to get a room, and later that day, I was brought to the doctor. When he walked into the room, I was white as a sheet and doubled over as I sat in a wheelchair. He examined me and asked me if I suffered from indigestion.

"No," I answered. "I have never had that issue."

"Well, it sounds like indigestion to me."

I gave him a puzzled look. "Are you serious? My pain is low in my pelvis. It happens on a cyclical basis. I know it's gynecological. It must be."

"No, it's just indigestion," he insisted. He left the room and came back with prescriptions for an antacid and a pain pill.

"This will help," he said. I didn't say anything else at that point. It was a waste of my time, and I didn't have the energy to argue with him. I just wanted those pain pills so I could get on that plane and get home. I knew those pain pills would just make me sleep through the trip.

Back in the room, my husband made several phone calls to reschedule our flight. I could tell from his demeanor that he was displeased that he had to do this.

***

Several months after returning from Las Vegas, the gossip at my job had become unendurable. I just could not take it anymore. I became very depressed and wanted to quit.

"Well, if you quit, then your next employer is going to wonder why you had a lapse in employment. That isn't going to look good on your resume," said my husband.

"Well, I would just tell them that I was sick," I said.

"Still, it wouldn't look good. Employers look at things like that with suspicion. It just isn't a good idea."

> **_Note_: Moradi et al. (2014) reported that employment was negatively affected by the endometriosis patients in their study. The impacts included:**
>
> - **Choosing part-time work**
> - **Leaving a job that they loved**
> - **Loss of promotion**
> - **Becoming less productive**
>
> **The researchers also noted that some were forced to go to work despite their severe symptoms because they were unable to get time off work. Non-**

compassionate bosses played into the negative experiences as they were worried about losing their job.

I became terrified to quit my job. My husband made it sound like any lapse in employment would end my career, and I certainly didn't want that. Of course, now I know that is not true, but at the time, I was young, and I believed everything my husband told me. So, I continued to push on and stay at my job. However, several months later, I was on the verge of a nervous breakdown, and I knew I had to do something. My husband just got a new job in northern Virginia, and we knew we were going to move out of state soon.

"We know we are going to move soon, so I would have to quit anyway," I said to my husband.

"Well, that's true," he responded.

"So why don't I just resign now so I can focus on my health before we move?"

He sighed. "Yeah, I guess that's OK."

I knew he wasn't happy with my decision. I could tell by the hesitation in his voice.

"Look, it will give me some time to rest and see if I can find the underlying cause of this. Future employers can't hold a move out of state against me, right?"

"Nope," he said as he just stood there, staring at me. There was very little support for me or my situation, and that was evident in his tone of disapproval.

Even though I knew he wasn't completely on board, I resigned the next day. I felt a load of stress come off me after I did this. However, when I went home that day and told my husband, I felt anxiety swell up in me again. I knew he didn't approve of my decision. I knew he wanted me to continue to work even through all the pain. It really hurt my feelings. I felt like I had no one to lean on as I traveled down this lonely road.

***

I did not know where to turn for help. I finally realized that if I wanted to see any change in this pattern of pain, I needed to help myself by doing my own research.

I started to read about nutrition. I had never really thought too much about what I ate during the day. As I read up on nutrition, I came to realize how poor my food choices had been over the years. I ate a lot of processed food and little fresh food. In addition, my husband and I would always look for food that was "no fat", thinking at the time that this was the healthy way to eat. Later, I realized that we couldn't have been more wrong.

> ***What we know today:*** **Today, we know that polyunsaturated fatty acids, such as omega-3 fatty acids, are vitally important for the proper functioning of the human body. Omega-3 fatty acids can be found in foods such as salmon, mackerel, herring, flaxseed, and fish oil.**

One day, my husband read an article in Prevention™ magazine about the health benefits of flaxseed. He walked into our bedroom, excited, and showed me the article.

"There are so many health benefits, and I am wondering if adding this to our food might help you. I mean it can't hurt, right?"

I sat down and read the article. I, too, was intrigued but a bit skeptical. Regardless, we ordered a bag of flaxseed, and we started sprinkling it onto anything we could – cereal, yogurt, spaghetti – just about anything. It was ground flaxseed, and it didn't have much of a flavor to it, so we couldn't even tell we added it. Several weeks later during my period, I noticed quite a dramatic drop in my pain levels. Was this coincidence, or was this a result of the flaxseed? Only time would tell.

I continued to do more research and dramatically changed my diet. At work, I began eating salads containing lettuce, shredded cheese, olives, broccoli, cauliflower, green peppers, banana peppers, cucumbers, red onions, and tomatoes. I would eat this for lunch for four to five days out of the week. We continued to sprinkle flaxseed on our food at home, and we started taking a daily fish oil supplement. I also took a daily multivitamin.

> ***What we know today:*** **Since I had such a great response to flaxseed, I decided to write a blog after my adenomyosis diagnosis post-hysterectomy in 2007 and suggested its use in the disorder. I also authored several books in which I touted the health benefits of using flaxseed. Since that time, there has been some concern over its use in estrogen-dependent disorders such as adenomyosis due to it being a phytoestrogen. This is a legitimate concern, and so I began to doubt flaxseed's effectiveness in adenomyosis. However, current studies have shown that flaxseed may actually be helpful in treating estrogen-dependent disorders. Refer to the section on flaxseed later in this book for more information.**

I changed my breakfast food from a bagel and cream cheese to a bowl of oatmeal. I routinely made baked salmon for two reasons: first, it is a major source of omega-3 fatty acids, and second, I was trying to eat fish at least once a week. I stopped buying white bread and instead bought multigrain or wheat bread for sandwiches. I discovered edamame and crab, and these foods quickly became two of my favorites; however, I eventually stopped eating edamame after my adenomyosis diagnosis as it contains soy which is contraindicated in those with estrogen-dependent disorders. I began to use olive oil in most of my recipes. I began to cook more, and I made a concerted effort to move away from processed food. I learned that lemon could help to detoxify the liver, so I started to add fresh lemon juice to my glasses of water.

Since I saw a notable decrease in my symptoms, I began to work toward a master's degree in Holistic Nutrition. I decided to do some further research into omega-3 fatty acids and irritable bowel syndrome which led to my thesis, "The Effects of Omega-3 Fatty Acids on Irritable Bowel Syndrome and Inflammatory Bowel Disease". I was so passionate about this thesis since it involved my own personal experience, and I am proud to say that the first draft was approved by the college.

Since diet did improve my symptoms, my husband suggested that if I worked out more, maybe my symptoms would improve even more. I decided to go with him to the gym. However, on my bad days, I found it extremely difficult to do this. He kept pushing me, so I went as much as I was able, but I resented him on those rough days as I knew he still had no inkling of what I endured each month with these attacks.

At this point, I was convinced that I did have irritable bowel syndrome and that my change in diet fixed the problem. But not so fast…the story continues…

***

That year, my husband and I went to see my family in Wisconsin over Christmas. My general practitioner had given me a prescription for Bentyl®, an antispasmodic that was supposed to stop or at least slow down the cramping pain that I was feeling during my attacks. On our first night there, we had a nice dinner and sat down to watch one of our favorite Christmas movies – Christmas Vacation with Chevy Chase. We had a wonderful time laughing through that crazy movie, but as soon as the movie ended, I started to get that bloated feeling again. I told my parents that I was going to bed, but by the time I got to the top of the stairs near the guest bedroom, I knew another attack was imminent. I headed to the bathroom and looked at my stomach. I looked about 3 months pregnant, and I started to feel that familiar pain. I quickly went to the bedroom, opened my suitcase, pulled out the bottle of Bentyl®, and took a pill. I returned to the bathroom and walked back and forth, hoping that this would help me to have a bowel movement. As the minutes passed, the cramping pain worsened, and it didn't take long for it to progress to severe levels. As I endured the pain, I waited and waited for the Bentyl® to kick in, but it never did. The attack proceeded as if I had not taken any medication at all!

This all took place as my parents and husband were getting ready for bed. My mom knocked on the bathroom door and asked if I was all right.

"No," I responded. "It's happening again."

She opened the door only to see me sweating, white as a sheet.

"What can I do?" she asked, the concern evident in her voice.

"Nothing. I just have to wait this out."

"Oh, you poor thing," she responded.

"I was hoping the Bentyl® would work, but it's not doing anything," I said, doubled over in pain.

I walked over to the guest bedroom where we were staying, clutching my stomach. My husband was already in bed.

"I am sick again," I said to him. He looked up at me with a worried look but didn't say much.

I went back to the bathroom and told my mom to go to bed. There was nothing anyone could do. I just had to endure it until it let up.

The next few hours were pure hell. It started off with severe bloating, severe cramping pain with horrible constipation. I nearly fainted several times, and sweat dripped down my face.

After a couple of hours of this, I became very nauseated. Suddenly, I felt like I needed to have a bowel movement. I sat on the toilet, but as soon as I pushed, I felt like I was going to vomit. I stood up, raised the toilet lid, and positioned myself to vomit. Then I felt like I was about to have diarrhea. I put the lid down and sat back down. I pushed but then felt like I was going to vomit again. I grabbed the trash can, and I had a horrible case of diarrhea while I vomited into the trash can at the same time.

I opened the bathroom door and whispered into my parent's bedroom.

"Mom? Mom?"

"Yeah, what's wrong?" she whispered back.

"I need some help."

She walked out into the hallway, and I told her what had happened.

"I am so sorry, but I vomited into the trash can."

"That's OK. Give it here," she said as she reached out her hand.

"I'm so sorry."

"You can't help it," she responded. "It's OK. I'll go take care of this."

"Thanks, mom."

I had a few more bouts of diarrhea before the attack slowly ended. I look back on this now, and it is very telling that I asked my mom for help and not my husband. Subconsciously, I knew who cared about me and my condition, and it wasn't my husband.

> ***Note:*** **After much research, I am at a loss for why these anticholinergic drugs did not work in my case. These drugs relax smooth muscle (the uterine muscle**

and the intestines are smooth muscle). These drugs should have worked.

***

Two days later, I was feeling a bit better even though I was weak because I was afraid to eat too much. We all decided to go shopping and enjoy the Christmas season. While we were out walking about, I started to talk to my mom about my health concerns.

"I am so sick of not knowing what is causing these attacks."

"I can only imagine. I wish I could do something."

"You know, at this point, I wish they would just find cancer."

"Oh, you don't mean that."

"Yes, I do! At least I would have an answer."

"But you don't want cancer," she replied.

"No, but I would have an answer."

My mom meant well, but even she did not fully understand what I was feeling at that moment. Harsh as it sounds, I really would have felt so much better at that point if the doctors had found cancer. Not only would I have a solid answer for my pain, but an actual diagnosis would possibly change the attitude of my husband's family, my co-workers, and friends who did not think anything was wrong with me. At the very least, it would relieve a truckload of the stress that was coming at me from every direction. I just wanted an answer.

Virginia (1997 – 2003)

1997

"Suffering should not define you as a woman, and just because you're a man it doesn't mean that it doesn't affect you! HELP HER to remove the taboos and the loneliness surrounding this disease; be understanding, show empathy, and don't accuse her of being sensitive, delicate, or overly dramatic – this is a big opportunity for you guys to show that you care and to be a real man!"

-Susan Sarandon

In 1997, my husband and I moved to the northern Virginia area. Although the attacks of severe abdominal pain were better, I still was having milder versions of the attacks. My stomach still bloated up markedly at the end of my period, and I still had dysfunctional uterine bleeding. Although diet changes clearly helped me, I strongly believed the root cause of the problem still had not been addressed. To make our move easier, I went back on Orthocyclen® during this time.

My husband seemed OK that I was going back on birth control pills. We had tried for so long without a positive pregnancy test, and I think both of us were exhausted and fed up. We both needed a break from the mental stress of it, and I think both of us just wanted me to feel good so we could enjoy life, especially vacations. However, my mother-in-law continued to put pressure on us to have children.

"The two of you would make such great parents," she said.

"Yes, but…"

"No, seriously. You two need children," she responded. "You will regret it once you get older if you don't have children."

"We have been trying," I said. "I just am not getting pregnant. My health issues…"

"Well, you just need to keep trying. Try A LOT! You're getting older, and you need to get serious about this."

I just nodded in agreement. She wasn't hearing me. It's as if she didn't want to believe that I had anything wrong with me. She was in denial, and I was invisible to her.

1998

"You wake up every morning to fight the same demons that left you so tired the night before, and that, my love, is bravery."

-unknown

A few months after our move, I saw a gynecologist in the area near our home. My blood work was normal (including a normal prolactin level), and a sonogram was done. A possible fibroid was noted on the scan.

***

After being at my new job for a little less than a year, I opened up to a couple of my co-workers who had become good friends. I only spoke to a few of them that I felt I could trust. I learned my lesson from my experience in South Carolina, and I made sure to be very selective as to who I spoke to about my issues. They told me about some highly ranked doctors in the area, and I decided to call and get an appointment with one of them.

In October, at my first appointment with this new female internist, I explained to her that I had a history of left-sided abdominal pain associated with my period accompanied by sweating, shakiness, nausea, vomiting, constipation, diarrhea, and a fast heart rate. I told her that the pain usually occurred at the end of my period when I was spotting, and that I had heavy periods that lasted anywhere from 10 to 14 days. At that time, I was on Orthocyclen® birth control pill, Bentyl® for abdominal cramping, and folate for anemia. I was 33 years old during this first visit with her.

I was happy with this internist as she listened attentively and seemed to be genuinely concerned. After discussing my medical history at length, she was also at a loss for what was wrong with me, but she assured me that she would do everything she could to help me. She decided to change my birth control pill to Ortho Novum 777®. She also ordered some bloodwork. According to her notes,

> *"Unclear to me what is happening – episodic but regular attacks, clearly related to the menstrual cycle. Raised possibility of panic attacks perhaps triggered by hormone surges."*

Later in her notes, she wrote:

> *"Plan gyn evaluation, possible neuro/psych."*

This bothered me when I read it because I thought she might think it was all in my head. A psych evaluation? Anyway, she referred me to a highly ranked gynecologist in the area. I was hesitant about staying on birth control since my husband and I were trying to have children, but the quality of my life was so bad off the pills that I really did not have much of a choice.

I left the office that day feeling a little bit encouraged. Finally, I thought, I had found a doctor that was at least willing to listen and to do whatever she could to help me. I had not felt like that in years. Maybe I would finally find the underlying cause of this, and it would all end.

***

One day, on my way to work in bumper-to-bumper traffic on interstate 66 in northern Virginia, my stomach started to bloat again. I started to get dizzy and shaky, and my heart started to race.

"You have got to be kidding!" I thought to myself.

I became mildly nauseated, and indigestion set in. I knew this was a panic attack, so I tried to slow down my breathing and relax as I was in the middle of traffic and by myself. I desperately tried to move over to the right lane so I could exit the interstate.

I did manage to make it to work, and everything seemed to settle down once I was there. I called the internist that day and managed to get in to see her. She thought I had heartburn, so she prescribed Prilosec®, but I did not remain on that medication for long because I knew it was a panic attack, and I knew that these attacks would continue until we were able to figure out the root cause of my pain and bleeding. At that point, I think the doctors were just throwing anything out there to see if it stuck.

Her notes stated:

"Heartburn vs. gastritis vs. ulcer."

Medication facts: Prilosec®, also known as omeprazole, is a proton pump inhibitor that is used to decrease acid production in the stomach. It is used in the treatment of gastroesophageal reflux disease, also known as GERD.

***

The follow-up with the internist was a few weeks later. I found out the results from my lab work during this appointment. The bloodwork that she ordered included a complete blood panel (CMP), H. pylori, urine catecholamines, and vanillyandelic acid (VMA). One blood test showed that my 5-HIAA level was a little low. The rest of the tests were normal.

Note: VMA (vanillyandelic acid) is a breakdown product of epinephrine and norepinephrine. This test is typically elevated in catecholamine-secreting tumors such as neuroblastoma and pheochromocytoma. Symptoms of a pheochromocytoma include flushing, dizziness,

sweating, a fast heart rate, and anxiety. It is a hormone-secreting tumor in the adrenal gland (the adrenals sit on top of the kidneys).

5-HIAA is a substance formed by the breakdown of serotonin in the liver. Low levels are seen in depression, OCD, multiple sclerosis, and other abnormalities. My 5-HIAA level was 2 mg. over 24 hours. The normal level according to the testing laboratory was 3-15 mg. over 24 hours.

At that time, I was congested and struggling again with sinus issues. She put me on Claritin® for allergies and Biaxin® for a possible upper respiratory infection.

***Medication facts:* Biaxin®, also known as clarithromycin, is an antibiotic that is used for many types of infections including acute sinusitis.**

I had bloody diarrhea while using Biaxin®, so it was stopped, and I was switched to Levaquin®.

***Medication facts:* Levaquin®, also known as levofloxacin, is a quinoline antibiotic used to treat a variety of infections including acute bacterial sinusitis.**

***

One day during my period, I began to have the fierce cramping pain again. I laid on the bed, writhing in pain. At that time, our computer was on a table next to our bed. As I moaned in pain on the bed, my husband sat at the computer and surfed the internet. He could clearly see me in this condition, but he just ignored me. I really felt like he didn't believe me and that this was all a show. It was either that or he just didn't care. I started to feel like I had to somehow prove to him that I was sick. I didn't know it at the time, but now I realize that I was in a very dysfunctional relationship. I certainly deserved better treatment.

During this attack, I went to the bathroom and had a bowel movement. When I stood up, I realized that I had passed almost all blood. It frightened me to death! I almost passed out. I walked out of the bathroom in tears and told my husband what I saw.

I called my mom to let her know what happened, but she wasn't home. My dad could tell that I was upset, so he asked me what happened, and I told him. He tried so hard to calm me down. I could tell he was genuinely concerned, and he told me everything would be OK. Looking back, I realized I received far more support from my dad that day than I ever did from my husband.

The next day, my husband and I went to see the internist. I was in tears in her office. She performed a rectal exam and an occult blood test, and it came back positive for blood. She referred me to a gastroenterologist who performed another occult blood test which, again, was positive. As it turned out, I had hemorrhoids and an anal fissure.

The gastroenterologist asked me if I suffered from constipation. I explained the whole story to him. He advised me not to push as hard when defecating which disturbed me greatly. If I did not push hard, the severe pain would not stop. But now I cannot push hard because if I do, more hemorrhoids and possible anal fissures will form. I was in a no-win situation.

"Well, my advice is to eat more fiber and drink more water. I will also prescribe some nitroglycerin cream. This will relax the anal sphincter which will help it to heal faster."

"Blah, blah, blah," I thought to myself. I had been eating more fiber. I had been drinking truckloads of water since my days in South Carolina. Has it helped? Very little. I was getting so sick of doctors. Would anyone ever be able to help me??

I went to the pharmacy to pick up the nitroglycerin cream and went straight home to apply it to the inside of my anus. This was not a pleasant experience, but I knew I had to do it, so I just took in a deep breath and did it. I laid on my couch afterward to get some much-needed rest. About fifteen minutes after I laid down, I started to get a throbbing headache, so I reached over to the table and picked up the prescription pamphlet. As I read it, I became nauseous.

Suddenly, I felt like I was going to vomit. I ran to the bathroom and vomited into the toilet. I went back to my bed to lie down. As I lay there, I closed my eyes and made sure I didn't move my head because it was severely throbbing by that point. I never vomited again, but it took several hours to get rid of that pounding headache.

The next day, I looked at my prescription again. It was at that time that I noticed the percentage of nitroglycerin in that cream was not the percentage that my doctor ordered. In fact, I had applied 10 times more than I was supposed to apply!

"You have GOT to be kidding me!" I exclaimed.

"What?" asked my husband.

"Look at this," I responded as I showed him the paperwork. "They gave me a prescription that was 10 times stronger than what I should have gotten."

"Unbelievable," replied my husband. "Call the..."

"I am right now," I responded.

I immediately called the pharmacy and told them about the mistake. The pharmacist apologized repeatedly. I could not believe that after all I had been through medically, this had to happen to me too. I was so exasperated.

***

We had been living in an apartment temporarily while we waited for our new house to be built. Finally, the day came for us to move in. We were so excited! Everything went well with the move; however, shortly after moving in and before we were unpacked, my husband had to leave town on business. I was left with a half-unpacked house while I worked full-time. This did not bother me too much as I like to keep busy. However, my in-laws insisted they visit right after our move. Instead of giving us enough time to unpack, they decided to come immediately and get there right as my husband arrived home from his trip. My stress grew exponentially. I worked full time, and I had to make sure we had enough blankets, towels, sheets, cookware, etc. to make my in-laws comfortable during their stay. This meant that I had to finish unpacking by myself.

I worked from 11 a.m. to 7:30 p.m. during that time, so I would get up early, unpack and clean as much as I could, go to work, and come home and continue to unpack, do laundry, and prepare my home for visitors. I did all this while bleeding for about 12 days straight, passing multiple large blood clots during the day, and dealing with severe abdominal pain. I was utterly exhausted, and extremely moody. It is a good thing that my husband was away during that time.

When my in-laws and husband arrived, my house had been almost completely unpacked, and everything was set up for my in-laws to have a pleasant stay with us. Things didn't slow down during that first weekend as they all wanted to tour the Washington, DC area, so I was unable to get the rest that I so desperately needed. I never said anything to my in-laws about how exhausted I was because I had learned from previous experience that they just did not understand my predicament, and I knew that they didn't want to understand it. I just kept a smile on my face and endured all of this even though I had a powerful desire to just lay down and sleep. I became an expert at "faking it" to keep other people happy. I learned in later years that was not the right thing to do. I should have spoken up.

***

I had to wait for two months before I could get an appointment with the gynecologist because she was in such high demand. Although miffed, I agreed to wait because I wanted the best possible care. In the meantime, I still had attacks, so I returned to the internist with the same complaints. She noted some stomach rigidity; however, she ultimately diagnosed me with anxiety and panic attacks. She also recommended relaxation techniques such as yoga. I felt again that she thought this could all be partially in my head.

1999

"When accompanied by pelvic pain, painful periods, backache, painful intercourse, ovulation pain, leg pain or ache, it is much more likely that these symptoms are the result of endometriosis and not a GI issue at all."

-Dr. Ken Sinervo

My fibrocystic disease continued, and some months, I wished that I could have surgery to cut off my breasts. It felt like I was dragging around two huge pieces of lead. My previous gynecologists had mentioned that if I reduced my caffeine intake, my symptoms would improve. This explanation really didn't make a lot of sense to me, however, because I do not drink coffee. My only source of caffeine was chocolate. The important thing that didn't make sense was the fact that they always became extremely painful during PMS, and then they were not sore at other times during the month. If it were too much caffeine, wouldn't they be sore all the time?

Sinus issues continued to be a problem especially during PMS. It was more of an annoyance to me. The severe abdominal pain took center stage, and I was completely focused on that. It was only in later years that I made the connection between sinus issues and PMS/menstruation.

Intercourse was becoming increasingly painful. The pain occurred at all times at this point, not just during PMS. I have heard women with endometriosis describe intercourse as having a hot poker shoved up your vagina. That is exactly how intercourse felt for me. I did not tell my husband about it though. I had learned to bury things deep inside me. He did not seem sympathetic to my plight at all, and I was uncomfortable talking to him about this issue. So, I just kept my mouth shut. I thought that if I told him, he would just complain about it. I did mention a few times during sex that it hurt, but it didn't seem to matter to him. I just put up with it. I started to have a glass of wine before sex in order to help me relax and take the edge off the pain.

I finally had the first appointment with the gynecologist in January. After telling her my story, she performed a Pap smear and pelvic. My Pap and pelvic was painful yet again, but I put up with it because I was desperate for an answer to my problem. I was crushed when she told me that everything looked normal other than the fact that I had an "retroverted" and "levoverted" uterus. This means that my uterus was pulled toward the back and to the side. This was considered a normal variant and was not thought to pose any problems, so it was noted but not addressed any further.

The gynecologist ordered day 3 labs and recommended that I take 800 mg ibuprofen 4 times per day during my period as an antiprostaglandin therapy. This sounded eerily familiar to what the doctor in South Carolina told me. I could not help but wonder what this would do to my stomach. This is quite a bit of ibuprofen to take for 10-15 days of every month. I was worried, but she was supposed to be a great gynecologist, so I agreed to her recommendations. Her diagnoses for my condition were endometriosis and IBS.

Note: **There are several known positions of the uterus which can occur as a normal variant or be a result of adhesions from endometriosis as they may pull the uterus in certain directions. Also, pain from fibroid tumors in the uterus will be felt in different areas according to the position of the uterus. In anteversion, the uterus is tilted toward the front of the abdomen. As an example, pain from fibroids in an anteverted uterus is more likely to be felt in the**

front of the abdomen. Conversely, in retroversion where the uterus is tilted toward the back, pain from fibroids is more likely to be felt in the patient's back. An anteverted uterus is considered to be the normal position of the uterus.

During this appointment, I told her that my moodiness and depression were getting worse. She felt like I would be helped more by taking Sarafem® rather than Zoloft®, so she switched me to this new antidepressant.

> ***Medication facts:*** **Sarafem®, also known as fluoxetine or Prozac®, is a well-known antidepressant medication. It has also been used to treat major depressive disorder, premenstrual dysphoric disorder (PMDD), obsessive-compulsive disorder (OCD), and panic attacks. It works by increasing serotonin levels in the brain, and it is in the class of selective serotonin re-uptake inhibitors (SSRIs).**

The following is part of the letter that was sent from my gynecologist to my internist:

> *"[Since beginning Ortho Novum 777®], her periods are shorter with less cramping, but she still has episodes of severe lower abdominal pain lasting 24 to 72 hours. She has had her thyroid function tests and states that they are normal. She had a laparoscopy in 1996 which showed 'slight' endometriosis that was ablated by laser. She states that there were implants on her right ovary and uterus. She has had a pelvic ultrasound which apparently showed a small fibroid. At the time of her laparoscopy, a tubal insufflation showed that her tubes are open.*
>
> *My impressions are:*
>
> 1. *Episodic pelvic pain.*
> 2. *History of endometriosis.*

3. *History of spastic colon. I suspect that her endometriosis and her spastic colon have added to the effects of prostaglandin release at the time of her menstrual periods. I have recommended that she try an antiprostaglandin preventatively. I have given her a prescription for Motrin 800 mg t.i.d. starting on the very first day of her menses to see if blocking her prostaglandins may help.*

4. *Delayed conception. Since she has had the initial portions of the basic infertility work-up given her laparoscopy in1996, I have suggested that she and her husband [see a fertility doctor]. I have also asked her to return for day 3 lab work at the end of this menstrual cycle. She will have to contemplate whether she wants to stay on the oral contraceptive pills while evaluating her episodic pain or whether she wants to try to conceive again at this juncture. I have asked her to obtain a copy of the operative report, which should have been dictated at the time of her laparoscopy to see if we can evaluate the extent of her endometriosis. She will schedule a follow-up appointment in April to evaluate these things further."*

***

I went to the lab on day 3 of my menstrual cycle and had several tubes of blood drawn. The following tests were performed:

- Follicle stimulating hormone (FSH)
- Luteinizing hormone (LH)
- Prolactin
- DHEA sulfate
- Estradiol
- Amenorrhea profile
- Thyroid stimulating hormone (TSH)

***

One day while having one of the few fights we had during our marriage, my husband blurted out that he thought I was frigid. I will never forget that because it was like he just shoved a giant dagger into my heart. He had no idea what I was putting up with to make him happy.

I always like to be busy. However, it was becoming increasingly difficult to be on the move constantly while suffering from severe pain and heavy bleeding. Since I worked full-time, I really looked forward to sleeping in on the weekends. But after we moved into our new house, my husband and I started to work on our house and yard all weekend, and it started to feel like I never had time to rest. It was like I was just working seven days a week with no break. I finally had a talk with him and told him that I needed to get some rest, especially during my period.

"OK, that's fine," he responded.

"So, on the weekends, if we go out, let's get home early so we can get laundry done and clean, so we don't have to worry about that during the week."

"OK," he said while watching television.

I reached for the remote and turned the television off.

"What?" he asked.

"Listen to me," I responded. "This is a big problem for me."

"You don't want to go out as much on the weekend," he said. "That's what you want, right?"

"I don't mind doing stuff on the weekend," I said. "I just don't want to be out ALL weekend. I need to get stuff done around here."

"OK," he responded, clearly bothered. He grabbed the remote and turned the television back on.

I left the room feeling conflicted. My instinct told me that he "technically" heard what I said, but he really didn't understand what I said.

After that discussion, we continued to go out on the weekends, but we never seemed to return "early." The discussion made no difference. Nothing changed. We still worked from morning to night – shopping, working in the yard, decorating the house, etc. I still did laundry and cleaned during what little time I had on the weekends and during the week. I was completely worn out. I do not know how I had the energy to accomplish everything I did while dealing with profuse bleeding and severe pain.

***

In February, after another bout of severe abdominal pain, I returned to the internist and told her that the pain had happened again. By this time, I was so confused that I didn't know where to go – the internist or the gynecologist! She told me the same story – that it was a combination of endometriosis and IBS. Since I was having such a tough time, she suggested to take the Motrin three days BEFORE my period started. This meant I would take Motrin for two to two and a half weeks out of every month! She also recommended that I see a counselor for anxiety treatment.

***

In April, I returned to the gynecologist and received the results of my hormone testing. I was absolutely convinced that something would show up on these tests. How could I be in so much pain with normal hormone levels? I just knew that this was finally going to be the "ah-ha" moment.

Well, it wasn't. Totally confused, I listened as she read out the results which were all normal. How could my hormone levels be normal with all the pain I was in?

The following were the results:

- FSH – 8.1 mIU/ml (range 1.1-9.6 mIU/ml)
- LH – 4.8 mIU/ml (range 0.8-25.8 mIU/ml)
- Prolactin – 17.7 ng/ml (range 2.8-29.2 ng/ml)
- DHEA sulfate – 60 ug/dL (range 45-270 ug/dL)
- Estradiol – 54.3 pg/ml (range 19-83 pg/ml)
- TSH – 1.23 uIU/ml (range .35-5.50 uIU/ml)

Note: **The range for FSH, LH, and estradiol vary throughout the month. Since these were day 3 labs, the ranges above were what should be seen in the follicular phase of the menstrual cycle. The follicular phase is day 1 to day 14.**

Marcelle Pick (2013), an OB/gyn nurse practitioner, explains the importance of looking at hormonal balance rather than individual hormone levels in her book, *Is it Me or My Hormones?* For example, she explains that if you have a high-normal estrogen level and a low-normal progesterone level, your practitioner may tell you that you are "normal." However, if you look at the estrogen to progesterone ratio, it may be abnormal. It is extremely important to look at the ratio to get a clear picture of hormonal balance. She also talks about how practitioners look at too few hormones. Some hormones that are commonly ignored in dealing with female issues are cortisol, adrenaline, and insulin. Note that none of these hormones were tested in my case. Additionally, progesterone wasn't tested. If my progesterone level had been tested and was found to be low-normal, estrogen dominance may have been picked up if the ratio was calculated. All these hormones are intricately interrelated and should be evaluated in any workup for female menstrual issues. See Estrogen Dominance for more information.

"I am going to order a transvaginal ultrasound," she said. "Everything on your exam appears normal, but if there is an issue, we should be able to see it on ultrasound."

She explained to me that during a transvaginal ultrasound, a probe is inserted into the vagina. It is not like a regular ultrasound.

"Great," I thought. "Something else to stick in my vagina which I am sure will cause more pain."

"Your bladder will have to be full. You might be a little uncomfortable because of that."

"Uncomfortable?" I thought. "You think I am going to complain about a full bladder when I have this excruciating pain every month?"

Of course, I didn't share these thoughts with my gynecologist. I was just becoming so cynical. These doctors didn't seem to have one clue about the horrendous symptoms I experienced every month. And they were just too busy to notice. It seemed like I was on this assembly line, and they were just stamping me with a "Done" stamp and then moving me on down the line. It's like I was imperceptible to others. Would ANYONE slow down long enough to actually SEE me??

***

When I arrived at the imaging office, my bladder was full, but I could manage being uncomfortable for a brief period. However, they were a bit backed up. After waiting about 20 minutes, I went to the front desk.

"How much longer?" I asked.

"We'll get to you as soon as we can," replied the girl at the desk.

"My bladder is about to burst," I replied. "I don't know how much longer…"

"If you need to go, just go a little bit, and then stop the flow. That's the best I can tell you. We are moving as fast as we can."

She seemed put off that I told her that my bladder was full. Upset, I turned around and sat back down. I didn't dare try to go "a little bit." I knew once I started to urinate, there would be no stopping. I just sat there, distended and tense, hoping that I didn't urinate in the waiting room. They finally called me back, and I did manage to get the ultrasound done before I urinated. It was such a relief when the test was over, and I was able to relieve myself!

In addition to being uncomfortable due to my full bladder, I also found the test to be quite painful. I watched as she put a condom on this long slender probe after which she applied some KY Jelly to help with the insertion. She gently inserted it into my vagina. That part was alright, but then she had to manipulate the probe several times to get good images of my ovaries. When she pushed the probe to the side, I felt a great deal of burning type pain in my vagina. At one time, it almost felt like a tearing-type pain just like I felt during my pelvic exams.

> ***What we know today:*** **Today, it is possible to identify adenomyosis on MRI and transvaginal ultrasound, but it requires a sonographer who is trained in adenomyosis. More information on this topic can be found later in this book.**

***

In May, I returned to my gynecologist. Again, my pelvic exam was normal. She noted on my chart that I had a history of endometriosis but did nothing else to follow up on that. We discussed the pros and cons of in vitro fertilization, and I agreed that it would be a good idea if I had an in vitro fertilization (IVF) evaluation.

The transvaginal ultrasound came back normal. I was devastated. I still had these attacks, although not as bad since I had changed my diet, but my periods were getting heavier and clottier.

***

On a Saturday night, my husband and I met my former boss and her husband for dinner in downtown Washington, D.C. She was my boss in South Carolina, but she had accepted a position at the National Institutes of Health (NIH) years ago. Now that we lived close to each other, we wanted to catch up. I was so excited to see her and her husband, but bad luck intervened, and I was in the heaviest part of my period on the day of the dinner. I felt awful, but I really wanted to see them.

We went to a nice restaurant where I ordered paella. It looked so delicious when it came, and I was ready to dig in. Suddenly, I felt a gush of fluid, and I was afraid to move for fear I would leak all over my clothes. I kept smiling and talking, trying not to draw any attention to myself. I politely excused myself, saying I had to use the bathroom. I had a completely soaked pad with clots sitting on top of it that were the size of dimes. I became dizzy. How could I lose so much blood and still walk around? Shouldn't I be unconscious or something?

> ***Note***: **Moradi et al. (2014) reported that the women in their study worried "about wearing white pants, sitting on white couches, or sleeping on white mattresses."**

I changed my maxi pad, cleaned myself up, and returned to the table. I was a nervous wreck for the rest of the meal. I remember hearing only parts of the conversation because racing thoughts were going through my mind. What if another gush comes, and this time I am not so lucky? What if it gets all over my clothes? We are over an hour away from home. What if I bleed all over the chair or all over the car on the way home? I was a complete mess.

To make matters worse, I took about three or four bites of my paella, and I could not eat another bite. I was both full and nauseated. Here I was at this nice restaurant, and my hormones caused big appetite issues. I tried so hard to hold it together. I kept smiling and acting as if nothing was wrong, and I think I did fool everyone. I do not think anyone noticed a thing except that I was not very hungry. I took most of my paella home to eat the next day.

***

PMS symptoms continued to worsen. I started to have bouts of insomnia right before my period started. I would get moody and be feel very tired, but when I went to bed, I could not sleep. I stared at the ceiling and walls, continually turned over in bed trying to get comfortable, and I just could not fall asleep. I didn't get up because I needed to work the next day and I needed the sleep desperately. I kept trying to force myself to sleep. The weird thing about this insomnia is that I felt so tired when I went to bed, but once I was there, I could not fall asleep to save my life!

The brain fog during PMS continued to get worse. At other times of the month, I would be able to concentrate well at work and get a lot done. However, during PMS, I would catch myself making more mistakes. Thankfully, I would catch them before I gave my work to my boss, but I would get so frustrated with myself. I felt like I could not concentrate as well for some reason, and no matter how hard I tried, I just could not get out of this "fog" until my period began. I strongly suspected a hormone imbalance was causing this issue. Could it be the same hormone imbalance that I thought was causing all my pain and heavy bleeding?

***

My in-laws came to visit one week during the summer. Once again, my mother-in-law insisted that we have children.

"The two of you really need to have children! It would be such a shame if you didn't have any kids because both of you would be just wonderful parents," she said.

"I know, mom," replied my husband.

"I know," I said. "We have been trying."

"But you really should have them," she continued. "Listen, when you get older and you don't have kids, you will regret it. Don't wait too long."

I just smiled and said nothing. I knew that no matter how much I tried to explain what was happening with me, she would never understand. The one thing she did not even consider, though, is that I WAS dealing with the thought that I might never be able to have children, and it was already breaking my heart. I had already considered what it would be like to never have a child, and it was devastatingly painful. She increased the amount of emotional pain I was already dealing with because her only concern was for her to be a grandmother. She was not thinking about my emotional well-being at all. I became increasingly emotional and mentally exhausted when I had to deal with her.

***

One day while at the mall, I passed by a Claires® shop and noticed that they did ear piercing.

"Hey," I said to my husband. "I think I want to try and pierce my ears again." I had told him what happened to me in my teenage years.

"OK," he said. We walked into the store where I got my ears pierced for a second time.

The same thing happened. I was fine while I had the studs in my ears for the first month, but the first time I put costume jewelry in my ears, I broke out again with a very itchy rash. However, this time the rash was not as severe as the one I had when I was

16. Regardless, it was bad enough for me to stop wearing earrings once again. I was extremely disappointed.

***

My husband and I made the decision to try for a pregnancy once again. I stopped the pill, but many months of trying resulted in multiple negative pregnancy tests yet again.

I made an appointment with a fertility clinic near Washington, D.C. Obviously, I was extremely nervous about this visit. With all the pain I was in, I expected the testing and in vitro procedure to be extraordinarily painful. I really wanted a child, but could I endure the pain to get one? I was scared to death.

I walked into the clinic with my husband, and I shook as I sat there, waiting to be called back. When the nurse finally called us back, I took a deep breath, stood up, and walked into the clinic, hoping I would not faint from the fear. I walked into the fertility doctor's office, and we both sat in the chairs behind the large cherry desk. I scanned the room and noted the framed degrees on the wall. Oddly enough, I settled down a little as I realized that this doctor was highly educated. A few minutes later, a doctor walked in.

She introduced herself at which time my anxiety skyrocketed again. I was just an emotional wreck. She opened the file and looked at it as we waited. Finally, she began to speak, keeping her eyes on the file.

"So, it looks like you have tried for pregnancy for quite a few years. Is that right?"

"Yes," we both replied.

"No positive pregnancy tests?

"No," I responded.

119

"Have you done anything else to enhance your chances of getting pregnant?"

"Well, I tried laying with my legs up in the air after intercourse. I heard that might help."

"Hmm," she responded, still looking at the folder.

"Anything else?"

"No," we both responded.

She looked up at us. "Well, let's go over a couple of things first," she responded. "I see in your records that you have a genetic translocation."

"Yes," I responded. "I learned that I had that about 15 years ago when I worked in South Carolina."

"What chromosomes are involved?"

"1 and 15," I responded. "And it's a fairly large translocation."

"Hmm," she responded. "Do you know they breakpoints?"

"Not off the top of my head," I responded. "But I do know that my risk of miscarriage is high due to the size of the translocation."

"Would you please get a copy of the karyotype and send it to me?"

"Sure," I responded.

"OK, she said. "Well, the first thing we should do is to run some tests on both of you." She looked at my husband first.

"We will need to run some tests on you to check the health of your sperm." She looked at me. "And we will need to check your hormone levels. You have already had a transvaginal ultrasound which was normal, so we don't need to repeat that."

"OK," we both responded.

The fertility doctor pulled out her prescription pad and wrote orders for a sperm test for my husband and a hormone test for me.

"Make a follow-up appointment with the front desk for about two weeks. We will discuss the results then and then plan our next steps."

We nodded as we took the orders from her. We made our next appointment, and then left.

***

A family that was close to us in South Carolina decided to visit us one weekend. We spent Friday night reminiscing about our fun times in South Carolina after which we all went to dinner.

The next morning, we all got up and ate breakfast together. At the time, my period was about 3 days late. I was hoping that this would be the month that I found out I was pregnant.

"What is up with you?" my friend asked.

I smiled. "I am 3 days late."

"What?" she asked. "Are you really?"

"Yes," I said.

The rest of the group overheard the conversation and listened intently.

"I have a pregnancy test," I said.

"Well, what are you waiting for?" asked my other friend.

I ran upstairs to get the test from my bathroom. I was so excited! What if I was pregnant, and my friends were all there with me when we got the news?

When I walked back downstairs, I heard my husband say, "You're not pregnant."

I gave him a dirty look. "How do you know?"

"You're never pregnant."

I was quiet. I walked into the bathroom and felt like crying. Not only was his comment thoughtless, but to say that in front of our friends was so disrespectful to me.

I took the test, and I was extremely disappointed to see that the test was, in fact, negative once again. I walked out of the bathroom, and my friends knew what the result was just by looking at me.

***

A few weeks later, we returned to the fertility clinic for a follow-up.

"Well, it looks like you have a uterine infection," said the fertility doctor.

"What?" I asked.

"There was heavy growth of E. Coli on your sample," she said.

"Really? Could that be causing my issues?" I asked.

"Well, no, probably not, but we have to get that cleared up before we do anything else. But everything else looks good."

"So, what do we need to do?" I asked.

"I am going to put you on Cipro® to clear the infection. Once that is cleared up, I want to put you on a fertility drug called Clomid®. I would like to try this for about six months or so. This may be all you need to do. But, if it does not work after about 6 months, we will start to talk about IVF." She took out her prescription pad and scribbled on it as I asked her some questions.

Medication facts: Clomid®, also known as clomiphene, induces ovulation by binding to estrogen receptors. This tricks the body into thinking estrogen levels are low. As a result, there is a surge in the levels of follicle stimulating hormone (FSH) and luteinizing hormone (LH). This triggers ovulation. This drug is used to treat female infertility. The following are possible side effects of using Clomid®:

- Nausea
- Vomiting
- Diarrhea
- Flushing (hot flashes)
- Breast tenderness
- Abnormal vaginal bleeding
- Headache
- Fatigue
- Vaginal dryness
- Blurred vision
- Depression

Use of this drug can result in multiple births. Additionally, Clomid® is listed as a category X drug, meaning that this drug is known to cause birth defects. Contraindications for the use of Clomid® include:

- Undiagnosed vaginal bleeding
- Endometriosis
- Uterine fibroids

Note: After researching Clomid® for this book, I wonder why I was prescribed this medication as I had a contraindication for use of this drug, namely endometriosis.

"Does this have any side effects?"

"Yes. You can expect to be a little moody, and it may make you a little nauseated. You may also have some hot flashes."

"Another pill that sounds like it will increase my already horrendous symptoms," I thought. However, I somehow found the strength to endure it because I knew this pill may result in a child.

While I was on Clomid®, we traveled 9 hours to Ohio for my 8th grade class reunion and my best friend's wedding. I felt fine during the wedding and the first part of the reunion, but about an hour into the reunion, just when the dancing was about to start (I love to dance), I suddenly had a massive hot flash followed by terrible nausea. I had to leave. I was so incredibly disappointed that I could not spend the evening having fun with friends that I had not seen in over 15 years.

I took Clomid® for the 6 months, and yes, my moods worsened. I was also nauseated from time to time and suffered from horrible headaches. After enduring all these difficult symptoms, I still was unable to get pregnant. Each time I took a pregnancy test and looked at the negative result on the test, my heart sank.

> ***Note***: **Moradi et al. (2014) reported that the patients in their study said they experienced a reduction in social activity due to endometriosis. They decided to stay home due to excessive bleeding, severe pain, and fatigue.**

***

After 6 months, we returned to the fertility doctor and told her that the Clomid was not effective since I did not get pregnant.

"So, we can move forward with IVF?" I asked.

"Yes, let's talk about that. OK, the risk of miscarriage is high since you have a large translocation. I think we would need to implant about 8 fertilized eggs. The reason I want to implant so many is because I am assuming about half of those would not be viable due to your translocation. So, that would leave four viable fertilized eggs, and I would expect that either one or possibly two of the viable eggs would attach to the wall of the uterus and progress to the formation of a fetus."

"Wow," I responded. I thought for a few seconds and. "But I understand that in theory, that's what would happen, but what if it happens that all the fertilized eggs were viable and say, six of them attached and I ended up pregnant with six babies?"

"Oh, I would never allow a pregnancy with six babies to continue. That is too dangerous. I doubt that would happen, but if it did, I would send you up to Philadelphia for selective termination."

"Like abortion?"

"Yes, but we would only abort a couple of them to make the pregnancy safer for you."

I looked at my husband and nodded my head. "No," I responded. "No, I can't do that. I can't kill my own baby."

A scowl came across the fertility doctor's face. She sat back in her chair in disgust. "Well, if you aren't open to that possibility, I can't help you."

Troubled, I stood up. "OK, well thank you for your time." I turned around and left the office. My husband did not say anything as he turned around and followed me out the door.

"I can't do that," I whispered to him as we walked out of the office.

"I know," he replied.

> ***What we know today:*** **I am so glad that we didn't waste our money on IVF at that time. Today we know that IVF fails quite often in patient with**

adenomyosis. Since I had no idea that I had adenomyosis at the time, we would have probably had a failed IVF attempt since I was not properly treated diagnosed.

My husband and I decided to let nature take its course. We prayed a lot and decided to leave it in God's hands. If God wanted us to have children, somehow it would happen. I went back on Ortho Novum 777® and managed my symptoms through this birth control pill, a healthy diet, and Motrin® as needed for pain.

***

Since IVF was now off the table, we discussed adoption.

"So today, I looked up some information about adoption," I told my husband as we sat down to have dinner.

"OK," he responded.

"There is a seminar in a couple of weeks that I would like to attend. Did you know we can do an open or a closed adoption?"

"What do you mean?"

"Well, I am not quite sure – I will get more info at the seminar – but from what I understand, a closed adoption means that there is no contact with the biological parent. An open adoption means the biological parent can interact with us and can have some limited contact with the child."

"Oh, definitely closed for me," he responded.

"You don't want to do an open adoption?"

"No," he said. "I worry that the parent would try to get the child back."

I looked at him and then looked back down at the papers in front of me. I took a bite of my food.

"So, what about adopting a child from someplace like China?"

My husband swallowed a bite of his food. "I don't know."

"No foreign adoption?"

He hesitated. "I don't know."

I stared at him for a few seconds. "I think an Asian child would be wonderful."

He remained silent as he ate his dinner.

"What's wrong?"

"I don't know. I really want a child of my own."

I put the papers down on the table. "So, you don't want to adopt?"

"I don't know."

"Then why am I doing this?"

He looked up. "It's good to get all the information. Just go to the seminar, and we will talk about it after you get back."

I looked down at the papers. "OK," I said quietly.

I did go to the seminar, and I was extremely interested in the adoption process. However, the cost really shocked me. This adoption process would eat up most of our savings, and I knew my husband would not be happy about that. On my way home, my instinct told me that adoption was not going to be the answer. I thought that if my husband wasn't 100 percent on board with this, it would be a bad idea to pursue it.

We did discuss it when I arrived home, but he still seemed hesitant about the entire process. He mentioned to me again that he really wanted his own biological child. Eventually, adoption discussions stopped, and I didn't push it. I didn't want to adopt a child with a husband who didn't support it completely. It would not be fair to the adopted child.

***

We went back to South Carolina for a visit with my in-laws. As we sat in the living room and talked, I suddenly felt a gush. I went to the bathroom where I saw that I needed to change my maxi pad as it was completely full. After urinating, I stood up and about a one-foot-long clot hung off me. I had to take a piece of toilet paper and pull it off. I had never seen a clot this large before, and it made me quite dizzy and shaky. I did some deep breathing, cleaned myself up, and got myself together. When I felt well enough, I walked back into the living room, sat down, and acted as if nothing was wrong. I was becoming an expert at putting on a happy face and not sharing the gory details of this demon that was wreaking havoc on my body.

***

PMS had become almost brutal for me. Eventually, I was diagnosed with premenstrual dysphoric disorder (PMDD).

> ***Note:*** **PMDD refers to a severe form of PMS that typically starts a week before a menstrual period and continue until a few days after a period starts. The depression, tension, and anxiety are worse than typical PMS. Symptoms include fatigue, severe anxiety, severe sadness or hopelessness, being "on edge," marked anger, food cravings, binge eating, bloating, breast tenderness, headaches, muscle pain, insomnia, severe mood swings, concentration problems, and suicidal thoughts.**

I did agree that I had PMDD. I hate to admit it, but I experienced all the above symptoms.

I remember one day when I was particularly moody. Thank goodness it was a Saturday. After my shower, I sat down in front of my bedroom window and cried for about thirty minutes. My husband even walked into the bedroom once and didn't say a word. I cried because I didn't know what was causing the pain. I cried because a lot of people around me thought I was making it up. I cried because my husband lacked compassion and understanding. I cried because the only empathetic person - my mom - lived halfway across the United States. I cried because I felt like a cow being moved along in a cattle herd when I went in to see my gynecologist. I cried because I felt infinitesimal.

Due to all the pain, PMS, heavy bleeding, hemorrhoids, and other symptoms, my sex drive tanked. I started to really dread having sex because of the pain. I think this low sex drive and that anxiety sex brought on just contributed to the overall problem. It probably increased my pain even more. I should have discussed this issue with my gynecologist, but I was too embarrassed to address it. I certainly did not feel comfortable discussing it with my husband after he told me that he thought I was frigid, so I just kept it to myself.

***

Hemorrhoids had become a persistent problem. I would use Preparation H® which would help short-term, but the pain and occasional bleeding would reoccur, so I returned to my internist who performed a rectal exam. She told me to increase my Metamucil intake and prescribed Anusol HC®.

> ***Medication facts:* Anusol HC® is a hydrocortisone cream that is used to treat pain, itching, and swelling of hemorrhoids in the anus.**

***

Another night and another attack. Once again, I woke up to searing pain across my lower abdomen. It was the same old story – quietly get out of bed and go to the other bedroom as to not wake up my husband. I endured three to four hours of wave-like pain that doubled me over. The same constipation occurred for several hours, and then diarrhea occurred which finally gave me some relief. Utter exhaustion lasted the whole next day.

That morning, after my husband got out of bed, I told him that I needed to go to the hospital. I wanted to be seen right after an attack. I thought that my blood work would be abnormal because an attack had just occurred.

"Do you really have to go?" he asked.

"Yes, I really do."

"Whenever we see the doctors, they always say you are OK."

"Listen, I really need to go. Last night was awful!"

He sighed. "Alright," he responded with a clear tone of irritation in his voice. We didn't speak during that trip to the hospital. Sadly, nothing was found while at the emergency room. All the tests that were run were normal.

***

In December, I started to get allergy shots again. The following is a portion of the initial report from my allergist:

> *History of present illness: This is a 34-year-old female who presents with the following history:*
>
> *Chronic nasal problems: Patient complains of nasal congestion, rhinorrhea, sneezing and postnasal drainage along with itching, watering, and redness of eyes on occasion. Symptoms are perennial and are persistent with seasonal exacerbation in spring and fall. Symptoms have been present more than 10 years. Exacerbating factors include pollen, cats, dust, grass, raking leaves, and change in temperature. She has tried over the counter decongestants which have helped, and Claritin®, which did not provide any relief. She has been tested for allergy in the past and was found to be sensitive to trees,*

grasses, weeds, and animal dander. She was previously on immunotherapy from 1994-1997 with improvement of her symptoms.

Chest symptoms: Patient has had wheezing in the past but has not had any episodes since beginning immunotherapy.

Atopic history: Significant for allergy to sulfa and penicillin. Patient has had hives and eczema in the past. Denies any atopic history of food or insect sting induced allergic problems.

Family history: Significant for allergy and asthma in her maternal grandmother, and allergy in her brother and mother.

Physical examination: The nasal septum is midline. Nasal mucosa appears edematous, boggy, and pale. No polyps are seen, and no sinus tenderness is noted. The tympanic membranes are normal bilaterally. No cervical lymphadenopathy is noted. Lungs are clear on auscultation.

Skin test results: Is markedly allergic to pollens of trees and weeds. Also is allergic to perennial allergen of cat. Mold allergy is also seen.

Assessment:

1. *Seasonal allergic rhinitis*
2. *Perennial allergic rhinitis*

Plan:

1. *Because of inadequate response to medication and significant allergy to items which are not avoidable, I think long term benefit can be derived from a course of immunotherapy.*

2. *An Epi-Pen® is to be kept on hand and used only as needed if symptoms of chest tightness, wheezing, urticaria, laryngeal symptoms or other systemic reactions occur.*
3. *Continue OTC decongestant.*
4. *Nasonex®, 2 sprays each nostril once daily.*

2000

"They're told it's all in their head. As a result, they can lose confidence and turn inward and get withdrawn and depressed."

-Dr. Tamer Seckin

In March 2000, a friend of mine told me about a condition called celiac sprue. Since I had been affected for so long with the gastrointestinal issues, she suggested that I might want to be tested for this condition. I made an appointment with the internist and discussed this with her.

> *Note:* **Celiac sprue is a digestive disorder where the patient is unable to process a substance in foods called gluten. Gluten is a protein that is found in wheat, barley, and rye. This substance causes inflammation in the small intestine and can prevent absorption of nutrients in food. Symptoms of celiac sprue are diarrhea, bloating, gas, and fatigue.**

Although I wondered if this was the issue, it was weird that it only flared during my menstrual cycle. However, I didn't ignore this possibility because I saw such a dramatic decrease in my symptoms when I changed my diet. I was desperate for anything to explain my symptoms, so I was open to ANY possibility, even if it didn't completely make sense.

The internist was hesitant to test me for celiac sprue, but she did order the test. However, the results were negative. It was a bittersweet moment as I didn't have celiac sprue so I could continue to eat anything I wanted, but I still did not have an answer to the cause of my severe abdominal pain.

***

I returned to my internist with another sinus infection. She thought it was allergies, but testing showed that I had a staph infection. I was put on Cipro® yet again. She also ran a CMP, cardiac risk profile, and a ferritin test. They all came back in the normal range.

I talked to her about my horrible headaches that happened during PMS. We discussed how I had light sensitivity during that time and the severity of the headaches. She thought that I might be having PMS migraines, so she gave me a prescription of Imitrex®.

> ***Medication facts:*** **Imitrex®, also known as sumatriptan, is in the class of selective serotonin receptor agonist class of drugs. It is used in the treatment of migraine headaches by narrowing the blood vessels in the brain. Side effects include drowsiness, dizziness, nausea, vomiting, diarrhea, flushing, tingling, and muscle cramps.**

***

Several months later, I returned to my gynecologist with the same complaints. I told her that I was having PMS migraines, light sensitivity, bad cramping, and large clots during my period. Motrin was helping very little. She performed a Pap and pelvic exam and stated that everything appeared normal.

"How can it be normal?" I asked. "I am bleeding up to 14 days straight. I get so bloated, and the pain is unbearable at times. How is that normal?"

She sighed. "Well, the next thing we can do is an endometrial biopsy."

She turned around, grabbed a pamphlet from a plastic container on the wall, and handed it to me.

"You can read that, and we can discuss it at our next appointment. But let me just tell you – an endometrial biopsy can be quite painful. So, think about that before you agree to do it."

Her tone and demeanor suggested to me that she didn't think an endometrial biopsy was necessary. It was as if she was saying to me, "If you keep complaining, we are going to do very painful procedures." I left totally disgusted. As soon as I got in my car, tears started running down my cheeks. I couldn't control my emotions.

"Stupid son of a bitch!" I blurted out. "Why the hell can't these idiots listen to me?" I jerked my seatbelt forward and forcefully locked it into place as I started to sob.

***

I felt like I was on an assembly line each time I entered the gynecologist's office. It was like I was being pushed through as fast as possible – do the exam, sign the chart, next, and on and on. I felt like the goal was not really to help me to get better, but to just push through as many patients as possible. It seemed like a race to see how many patients she could see in one day – like she was trying to break her previous record. It seemed clear to me that she did not want to be "bogged down" by difficult patients or cases. Since things were so rushed, there really wasn't enough time to get her to really understand what was going on with me.

I continued to complain to my gynecologist about my symptoms even though she "threatened" me with an endometrial biopsy. The next time I had an appointment, I decided to be completely prepared. I sat down at my desk and wrote out a list of my symptoms:

1. *Severe moodiness – uncontrollable crying*
2. *Extremely bad depression – feeling out of control, can't deal with stress, feeling overwhelmed*
3. *Severe breast pain in left breast only - normal exam and mammogram except for fibrocystic disease*
4. *Insomnia during PMS – some nights only getting 2 to 3 hours of sleep*

5. *Horrible headaches – possible migraines, have Imitrex*
6. *Heartbeat problems – feeling like it skips a beat and getting dizzy/lightheaded*
7. *Extreme appetite fluctuations – sometimes there is near constant hunger, other times no appetite and nausea*
8. *Extreme fatigue – unable to concentrate*
9. *Excessive urination*
10. *Shakiness*

When she walked into the exam room, I immediately told her that I had written all my symptoms down on a sheet of paper and that I wanted to discuss them with her.

"Go ahead," she said as she fiddled through my chart. I started to describe each symptom to her; however, she never looked up from the chart. I was about halfway through the list when she finally stood up and told me to lie down.

"But, I have more…"

She grabbed the paper from my hand, quickly glanced at it, and tossed it on the chair. She sat down on her stool, told me to relax, and began her exam.

I was devastated. What would it take for a doctor to listen to me? Really listen? It was clear to me at that point that she just wanted to quickly do my exam and then move on to the next patient. I endured the pain of the pelvic exam as I always did, but this time, I was also completely enraged. The fury inside me almost made the pelvic exam bearable because my mind wasn't so focused on the exam but on the strong urge to sit up and smack the crap out of her.

Once the exam was over, I sat up and spoke up again about my symptoms as she scribbled out a script for more bloodwork.

"Wait…I have more questions," I said.

"Hurry up. I have lots of other naked women waiting on me," she responded as she headed for the door.

I pushed my emotions down as far as I could. I knew that if I provoked her any more than I already had, she wouldn't help me at all.

"What about all of my symptoms?"

"Let's just wait for the results of your Pap and bloodwork. Right now, everything appears to be normal, OK?" she replied as she opened the door and exited the room.

Normal. I was so damn sick of that word. How can things be normal when I was experiencing so much pain each month? I once again remembered my ruptured appendix and what my uncle said:

> *"This could have killed you. Never put off getting medical attention if you ever feel pain like that again!"*

I knew the pain wasn't normal, and I knew I had to keep fighting, but at that point, I never wanted to see this gynecologist again. I felt like I was in the deepest valley of my life, screaming for help, and no one would listen. The feeling of invisibility was enveloping me like a dark cloud, and there was no way out. I was utterly alone in this.

> ***Note*: In a study by Moradi et al. (2014), the researchers stated some of the endometriosis patients had negative experiences with their physician "who did not want to listen to their concerns, had no time to answer their questions, and told them that the symptoms they experienced were 'normal' and 'not serious.'" One patient stated, "I went to a specialist in Sydney. I had a lot of questions and thought that because he is a specialist having to deal with hundreds and hundreds of people that he can give me**

the answers to my questions, but he did not have time to talk.”

I took the bloodwork script to the lab and once again had my blood drawn, but I expected the results to be normal as usual. was so sick of wasting time doing the same tests over and over again.

***

Several months later, I had the worst attack in five years. I had five bouts of diarrhea in two hours after suffering through several hours of severe constipation. At the next appointment with my internist, we discussed IBS vs. constipation, and she recommended that I use Dulcolax®, Fleet® enemas, magnesium citrate, Bentyl®, and prune juice to manage my constipation.

That Christmas was challenging for me as I love to indulge in Christmas cookies and especially chocolate. However, I really wanted to stay away from sugar because the reduction of sugar in my diet helped me a bit. Also, I wanted to try the whole “cutting out caffeine” thing to help reduce my fibrocystic disease symptoms even though I had my doubts. I asked my husband to tell his parents to please not send chocolate that year. I knew if chocolate was in the house, I would eat it. I am just not strong enough to turn it down if it is right in front of me. This “no sugar” thing was extraordinarily difficult for me. He did tell his parents this, and I felt relieved.

About a week before Christmas, we received a package of gifts from my in-laws. When we opened the box, there were wrapped gifts and two stockings. We opened all the gifts first, and then we went through our stockings. Cute little items were on top, and we were really enjoying everything we received until we got to the bottom of our stockings. They were packed with Hershey’s® kisses!

“Really??” I exclaimed. “Didn’t you ask them not to send chocolate??”

"Yeah, I did," replied my husband.

"Then why did they send it??"

"I don't know," he replied.

I was livid. I could not believe that they did this. When my husband talked to them later that day, he asked them why they sent chocolate when we specifically asked them not to do that.

"Everyone needs a little chocolate on Christmas," my mother-in-law replied.

Again, I felt unseen and alone. I asked a simple favor from a relative, and what happened? She ignored me. Completely ignored me. I felt so exasperated and exhausted.

After Christmas, I did manage to stay away from chocolate for a while, but I saw no decrease in my fibrocystic disease symptoms. My gut told me that this breast pain was all due to a hormone imbalance. It's the only thing that made any sense to me.

2001

"Absence of evidence is not evidence of absence."

-Dugald Bell

In January, I had horrible breast pain along with severe abdominal pain. I decided to return to my internist. She noted that even though I had stopped my intake of caffeinated drinks and chocolate, the pain in my breasts worsened. She performed a breast exam and found masses in both breasts, so she ordered a mammogram and a pregnancy test. PMS and anxiety were the diagnoses that she assigned to me, and that irritated me so much. Anxiety again – like it's all in my head! She also told me to take calcium and magnesium supplements as this might help with my breast pain.

> *Note*: **In a study by Moradi et al. (2014), patients with endometriosis used the following words to describe their feelings in dealing with the disorder: upset, angry, uncertain, weak, powerless, helpless, hopeless, exhausted, defeated, frustrated, disappointed. They also felt like they were a burden to others.**

During this appointment, I also received the results of the bloodwork that was drawn the previous month. Everything was normal except for MPV which was elevated.

> *Note:* **MPV stands for mean platelet volume. It may be elevated in the following conditions: hyperthyroidism, vitamin D deficiency, stroke, high blood pressure, heart disease, diabetes, and certain cancers. Additionally, recent studies have suggested that MPV may be elevated in adenomyosis. Increased MPV means that the platelets in the blood are larger than average, and this may be an indication that there are too many platelets in the blood. See section**

on platelet aggregation later in this book for more detailed information on this topic.

***

The yeast infections continued. I wondered if other women had this much of an issue with yeast. I knew that birth control pills could increase the risk of yeast infections, but this seemed excessive to me, and I was too shy to bring the topic up to even my closest friends. I was sick of constantly buying Monistat!

***

A few weeks later, the results of my mammogram came back. The following is an excerpt from the report:

> *Your patient had a low-dose screening mammogram. The breast tissue is extremely dense, which lowers the sensitivity of mammography. Benign-appearing calcifications are present in the left breast. However, no dominant mass, significant asymmetry, architectural distortion or clustered microcalcifications are demonstrated. There is no radiographic evidence of malignancy in either breast."*

In addition to getting the results of my mammogram, I had another sinus infection. I told my internist that I had been taking lots of Advil Cold and Sinus because that was the only thing that worked for me. It was as if I had to put a stick of dynamite up my nose to get it to drain. She told me that she thought it was allergies which I thought was peculiar since it was the middle of winter when I usually do not have allergy issues. She gave me a prescription for Astelin® spray.

Medication facts: **Astelin® spray is an intranasal antihistamine that treats allergic rhinitis.**

***

After this appointment, I went a while before going back to any doctor because I was so embittered with doctors in general. I was convinced that no one was going to be able to help me. My youthful attitude that doctors would always make me feel better had been crushed by this illness. I had never imagined that the doctors could not figure out the cause of my pain and profuse bleeding. These were doctors…they are supposed to be able to give me an answer.

Around this time, I started watching the TV show Mystery Diagnosis. I was intrigued by these stories because the patients had undergone a similar experience – they knew something was wrong with them, but their doctors kept telling them that they were fine. After many years of suffering, all the patients eventually got a correct diagnosis. Should I send in my story? Will that day ever come when I know what the problem is?

***

Another severe attack occurred again on another night. All I could do was pray.

"Please do not let me pass out, please don't let me pass out! Please get me through this, God!"

It was just me and God. My husband was asleep in bed, completely oblivious to the hell I was going through that night.

The attack finally stopped, and I went back to bed. When the alarm went off, I stayed in bed.

"Aren't you going to get up?" asked my husband.

"No, I am not going to work today. I had a horrible night."

He turned over and said nothing.

I called in sick to work and made an appointment with my internist. Later that day, I went to her office. When she opened the door to the exam room, she quickly noticed that I was in tears.

"I'm so sorry," she said in an empathetic voice. "I'm so sorry, but I'm still not sure what's going on here."

I could see the sympathy in her eyes, and I know she did care. I'm sure she was just as frustrated about this as I was.

I was once again told that I had IBS. I knew this diagnosis was wrong. First, I was told that IBS is a diagnosis of exclusion which means that all other known conditions have been ruled out, so they attach the term "IBS" to the problem. It basically means that "something is wrong, but we do not know what is causing it." This "diagnosis" just irked me even more. Second, these attacks kept happening at the end of my period. This MUST somehow be linked to my menstrual cycle. This MUST be a hormonal imbalance. What else could it be?

The internist gave me another prescription for Bentyl®. I left the office feeling like I just wasted an afternoon…and time off work…for nothing. I knew the Bentyl® wasn't going to work because it didn't do anything for me when I became so sick in Wisconsin. Since I had what felt like terrible constipation during the first half of the attack before I started to have diarrhea, she recommended again that I drink prune juice and take magnesium citrate to help regulate the function of my intestinal tract. I reluctantly agreed to do so, but I left the office extremely defeated.

***

The large blood clots that I passed during my period were occurring more frequently and had become exceptionally large just like the one I passed when visiting my in-laws in South Carolina. Migraine headaches became the norm for me during my period. I also noticed that I was feeling a great deal of pressure on my bladder during my period, and I was constantly running to the bathroom. I went in for yet another appointment with the internist.

I felt at this point that this doctor was getting a impatient with me. I kept coming back to her with the same complaints, but she never found a concrete reason why I was having so much trouble. She did not seem to want to spend as much time with me, and I felt very rushed to get through the appointment. Of course, she could have been having a bad day. Regardless, this only added to my agony.

I left the office that day with the diagnosis of menstrual migraines and another prescription for Imitrex. She also told me to monitor the frequency and size of my blood clots because if that problem continued, I would need an endometrial biopsy.

> ***Note***: **Sinaii et al. (2002) reported that 64% of women with endometriosis in their study stated that they had menstrual headaches compared to 45% of women without endometriosis that was reported in other studies.**

Great. She wants me to have that one test that my gynecologist "threatened" me with. A co-worker also mentioned to me that she had an endometrial biopsy, and it was excruciatingly painful for her. My stress level skyrocketed at the thought of having this done.

> ***Note***: **In general, an endometrial biopsy is not the best way to diagnose adenomyosis. Since the biopsy takes a sample from one or a few places inside the uterus, it is a matter of luck if the biopsy site has adenomyosis since it may not be present throughout the entire uterine wall. If a biopsy comes back negative, it does not rule out the presence of adenomyosis. Therefore, an endometrial biopsy is not recommended as an effective way to rule out adenomyosis. However, it can be effective at ruling**

out other causes of abnormal bleeding. For example, if there is concern for cancer, an endometrial biopsy may be highly effective. It all depends on what the physician is searching for in the patient.

***

One day at work, a coworker mentioned that she had heard remarkable things about a gynecologist in the area.

"Maybe you might have better luck if you went to him," she said.

"Maybe," I responded. "Do you have his info?"

"I'll get it for you and bring it in tomorrow."

"Wonderful! Thank you so much!"

After she gave his name to me, I called and made an appointment. I had to wait about a month to see him, but finally the day came. It was difficult for me to be optimistic, but I kept telling myself that maybe this time, I will get an answer.

He walked into the exam room, introduced himself, and took my medical history. He performed a Pap and pelvic exam which, once again, caused me great anxiety and pain; however, I just took deep breaths and somehow found the strength to get through it. When it was over, I felt so relieved.

"OK, your exam is normal, so let's just wait on the bloodwork. Schedule a follow-up with me in about two weeks, OK?"

"Alright," I responded as he opened the door and left the room. I couldn't help but feel a little disappointed. He just repeated the same tests that all my other gynecologists had done. Why should I expect different results? I just knew deep in my heart that he would not find anything else either.

Two weeks later, I returned for the follow-up. The nurse directed me to his office. I sat there waiting in front of a large desk. I scanned his walls and saw his medical school diploma proudly displayed on the wall behind his desk. Suddenly, he appeared and walked behind his desk, carrying a folder which, I assumed, to be my chart.

"So, your blood tests have all come back normal," he said.

"So, then what is wrong with me?" I asked.

"Let's review your symptoms again," he responded.

"I am having extremely heavy and prolonged menstrual bleeding, sometimes lasting up to 14 days. I am also passing large blood clots."

"OK," he said. "What else?"

"The pain is unbearable." I looked down at my hands as I tried to explain the pain as best as I could. "It usually hits me in the middle of the night for some reason, and it usually happens toward the end of my period. It comes in waves. I sweat like crazy, and I almost pass out from the pain. Sometimes I cannot even stand – I rock back and forth on my knees. If I did not know any better, I would think I am in labor…"

I looked up, and the gynecologist had his eyes closed. Was he sleeping?

"I just…can't take it…anymore," I said with hesitation. Should I continue? Should I just get up and leave? I just sat there, disturbed, as I knew deep down inside that this was just another waste of my time. I decided to stop talking to see if he would respond at all.

He struggled to open his eyes once he realized that I was not talking. I could clearly tell at that point that this man was completely exhausted and was not fully listening to me. He just wanted to sleep.

"Well, I don't see any issues on your exam or in your blood work." He looked down at my chart as he struggled to open his eyes. "Results of your bloodwork show that your TSH was 1.8, your FSH was 4.1, and your prolactin was 17.0 which are all normal. I think the best treatment course for you would be to continue birth control. A counselor might help you as well to help with your anxiety."

I was furious! Trying to be polite, I thanked him for his time and quickly left before I said anything I would regret. I returned to work.

"How did the appointment go?" asked my co-worker.

"Don't ask," I said. I was still fuming mad.

"Uh, oh," she responded. "What happened?"

"He literally fell asleep in front of me," I said as I shoved my purse into my desk drawer.

"What???" she asked in disbelief.

"I am not kidding. He fell asleep. Then he recommended that I see a counselor for my anxiety."

"No way!" she exclaimed.

"Yep."

"I am so sorry! I had heard some good things about him, but I guess I was wrong."

"Oh, it's not your fault. You didn't know him. You were just trying to help, and I really appreciate that."

"Still, I feel really bad."

"Seriously," I said, "no worries. I mean that. I'm just mad at him!"

***

"I've been up all night," I said to my husband. "I had another attack. The pain was intense. I swear sometimes I am having a miscarriage."

My husband didn't respond.

"I am exhausted," I said as I climbed into bed. Normally, it was time for me to get up and go to work, but there was no way I could on that day. I felt like I had been hit by a truck - complete and total exhaustion, a sore abdominal area from all the cramping, a burning anus from the diarrhea, and to top it all off, I was still bleeding.

"When are you getting up? I need to get in the shower soon."

I usually took the first shower because I had to be at work before my husband. Was he really asking if I was going to work? Didn't he hear a word I said?

"Didn't you hear me? I had a horrible night. I am calling in today. There is no way I can work in this condition."

My husband did not say a word. Instead, he got up, went to the bathroom, and took a shower. I felt like the biggest loser. I felt like he did not believe that I was in all this pain. Why didn't he believe me? Was I just a pathetically weak person for not being able to handle this pain?

In the later years, I found myself trying to "prove" to him that I was sick. I would give details of what I had endured, hoping that he would somehow understand the misery I had endured. He made me feel as if this pain was all in my head. After all, he is the one who suggested that I go on an antidepressant.

The way that my husband responded to my illness really made me feel as if I was the crazy one. His comments and lack of compassion broke down my self-esteem, and it was already damaged from other sources – my co-workers in South Carolina, my doctors, and my mother-in-law. I felt so alone. The invisibility of my disease had broken me.

I had become pessimistic. I covered up my anxiety, my fears, and my pain. I had become afraid to show how I truly felt for fear of rejection. I tried to make everyone around me comfortable and happy while "pushing down" my own feelings. It was easier that way...or so I thought. My favorite time of day was when I got in my car to drive home from work. I was able to listen to the music that I liked. I was able to set the car temperature to my liking. If I was freezing cold from bleeding too much, I could blast the heat without any complaints from my husband. For the few hours I had at home, I could sleep if I was exhausted, or I could sit down and really relax without having the pressure to make others happy. I really enjoyed being by myself during that time. I did not have to "act" like everything was perfect. I did not have to cover up my illness. Later in life, after years of counseling, I learned all about self-awareness, and I realized how I desperately lacked in self-awareness at that time in my life.

In the early part of 2001, I had another appointment with my gynecologist. I explained to her that my abdominal pain had continued unchanged along with my menstrual problems. Because of this, I was having a tough time with depression. She increased my dose of Prozac.

***

I went back to my gynecologist with complaints of rectal pain and bleeding. I was told to eat Metamucil® wafers during the luteal phase of my cycle. The luteal phase refers to the time from ovulation to the beginning of menstruation. I was very doubtful that this would work since I had been using Metamucil® for many years without any meaningful change in my symptoms. I was exasperated. She did, however, put me on a continuous dose of the birth control pill Yasmin®. This meant that I would only have four periods per year.

Medication facts: Yasmin® contains the progestin drospirenone and the synthetic estrogen ethinyl estradiol. It is a type of combination birth control pill.

***

I went back to my internist with sinusitis once again. This time she ordered a sinus x-ray to make sure there wasn't anything, such as a polyp, that would cause an obstruction in the sinuses. She told me to continue with the Astelin® spray and to start doing sinus rinses. The sinus x-ray came back negative.

***

Several weeks after starting on Yasmin®, I started to develop a crampy feeling in my right leg. At work, I would massage my leg and flex my right foot up to try and get it to stop cramping. After about a week of this, I started to do some research. I found out that this symptom might be a sign of deep vein thrombosis (DVT). I went back to see my gynecologist.

She came into the room, quickly looked at my leg, and determined that it was not DVT. She told me that she wasn't too concerned since my leg wasn't red or swollen. However, years later I learned that DVT was a major issue in women who had been on Yasmin®. In fact, lawsuits have been filed against the manufacturer regarding blood clots with this pill. Of note is the fact that the cramping pain in my right leg stopped once I stopped taking Yasmin®. Was this in fact a developing blood clot in my right leg? I will never know for sure, but I am suspicious even though my gynecologist wasn't concerned at the time.

Note: **Studies have shown that drospirenone, the active progestin in Yasmin® and some other birth control pills, is linked to an increased risk of blood clots. Additionally, Yasmin® may increase potassium levels in the body.**

153

In July, I had my routine Pap smear and pelvic exam which were, once again, normal. I had been eating Bran Buds® for several months, and it improved my symptoms a bit. It was around this time that I realized that I needed to drink a LOT of water when eating a high fiber diet. None of my other doctors had told me to increase my water intake when I increased my fiber intake. This shows a remarkably simple lack of communication and/or lack of nutritional knowledge by doctors. This little tidbit of knowledge could have made my life so much easier when dealing with these disorders as it may have reduced my constipation issue dramatically during that time.

***

My husband and I decided to take a trip to an outlet mall about an hour away from our house. It was Christmas, and we needed to do our Christmas shopping. After a full day of shopping, we stopped by Target® on our way home. As we walked through the store, I suddenly felt that all too familiar twinge of pain, and my stomach quickly became bloated. I knew I was in for another attack.

"We have to leave," I said.

"What? Why?"

I put my hand on my stomach. "My stomach. I can feel it, and I am bloating fast."

"We're almost done," he said. "Can't we just finish?"

"No," I insisted. "We have to leave now." I knew that when these symptoms started, I had very little time before they would get out of control. I knew the severe pain was only minutes away.

Exasperated, my husband followed me out of the store. By the time I arrived at the car, I was partially doubled over. I quickly got into the car and adjusted my seat to recline.

"Hurry," I said.

We started home, and I concentrated on my breathing. Slow, deep breaths, try to remain calm – that is all that I would allow myself to think. My husband was quiet all the way home. I knew he was not happy that he had to drive me all the way home without finishing our shopping trip.

Luckily, the pain never progressed to a full-blown attack that time. Even though my stomach had pouched out to about the size of a 4-month pregnancy and I had some moderate discomfort, I was just thankful that the pain had not progressed to the severe level that I was so used to at that time.

***

Eventually I started a new job at a large cytogenetics lab in Virginia. I worked predominately on cancer cases where I performed chromosome analyses. After about a year, I was nicknamed the "complex queen" because I always seemed to pick up complex cases in which the chromosomes had broken apart in many different pieces and into different rearrangements. These cases were like a puzzle. I downloaded pictures onto a computer screen, and I had to move the pieces of the chromosomes around to see if I could identify them. These kinds of cases were from those with advanced or terminal cancer, and they were exceedingly difficult. Those cases would exhaust someone who is healthy, but just imagine having to do that kind of work when you are gushing blood, cramping continuously,

155

and on many occasions suffering from a migraine headache. It was almost unbearable!

One day while working on a complex case and having my period at the same time, I was so tired that I was worried I would not be able to make it home. I got a Coca-Cola from the vending machine, got into my car, and began my 30–45-minute drive home. I remember closing my eyes at a stop light but opening them quickly because I felt myself drift off to sleep. It took just a few seconds. I did not do that again! Instead, I grabbed my Coke, drank it, and concentrated on keeping my eyes open all the way home. It was hard…a real struggle. When I finally arrived home, I walked in, dropped my purse on the kitchen table, went straight to the couch and was asleep in a matter of seconds. In fact, I hardly remember my head hitting the pillow. My husband woke me up when he arrived home. Dinner wasn't ready, but at that time, I do not remember him complaining; however, comments about not having dinner ready were made when this happened in later years.

***

Several months later, I had a particularly bad menstrual cycle. Symptoms included severe cramping, hot flashes, night sweats, vomiting, and passing blood clots. I was very hesitant about returning to my gynecologist, but I did anyway. During the exam, she said that there was a possibility that I had a fibroid present in the uterus which could be causing my problems. I was told to stop the birth control pill and start on Ponstel®, also known as mefenamic acid. She would see what effect this had on my menstrual cycle for two to three months and then decide if a surgical procedure would be necessary to remove the fibroid. I filled the prescription and began to take the medication.

Years later, I look back on this exam and wonder if she felt an adenomyoma instead of a fibroid. During those years, it was hard to tell the difference between a fibroid and an adenomyoma, and it is even difficult to do so today.

> *Medication facts:* **Ponstel® is a prescription NSAID. It is used to treat mild to moderate pain and is most often used to treat menstrual cramps. Side effects include bloating, constipation, diarrhea, dizziness, nervousness, heartburn, nausea, and ringing in the ears. This drug puts the patient at an increased risk for heart attack and stroke.**

> *Note:* **A fibroid tumor, also known as a leiomyoma, is a mass found in the uterine wall. It is a benign tumor, and estrogen has been shown to stimulate its growth.**

As you can see, the side effects of Ponstel® include constipation and diarrhea. Really? So let me get this straight – my most disabling symptom is severe pain due to constipation followed by diarrhea. Now she is giving me a pill that may cause constipation and diarrhea? How exactly does that make any sense?

I filled the prescription and began to take the medication; however, it was completely ineffective. During a follow-up visit, she stopped the Ponstel® and put me back on continuous Yasmin®. She decided to take a "wait and see" approach to the possible fibroid. So, for the umpteenth time, I was sent home with different medication in dim hopes that this time I would get some relief.

***

One afternoon, I cancelled plans again with our friends because I wasn't feeling well. My husband finally showed his true feelings about my physical health.

"You are always cancelling plans," he said.

"I am sick!" I exclaimed.

"You are always sick. You never feel good!" he retorted.

"I can't help this," I responded. "I thought you understood that."

"Look, even our friends are talking about how much you cancel plans," he said. "They are tired of it too."

"I can't help it," I said with tears in my eyes. "Do you really think I like the fact that I am in pain? Do you really think I like to cancel plans?"

He didn't respond.

> ***Note***: **Moradi et al. (2014) reported that study participants were frustrated about the unpredictability of endometriosis. One patient talked about how she couldn't plan events. She stated, "I want to plan something like a holiday, but I cannot plan it because you don't know what's going to happen... you are arranging your life around the disease. It controls you even if you don't want it to."**

"I am bleeding non-stop. I am in pain. I cannot do anything about it. The doctors sure as hell aren't helping me. What do you expect me to do?"

"Work out," he responded. "Go to the gym. Get in shape!"

"You know I have tried that," I responded.

"Not consistently," he said.

"I can't go consistently because of the pain!"

I started to cry out of sheer exasperation. He turned around and walked out of the room.

I felt utterly misunderstood and alone. I was completely invisible to him, to my friends, and to my doctors. I was utterly helpless and had no idea where to turn.

> ***Note***: **Moradi et al. (2014) reported that their study group stated that pain limited their normal physical activity. One patient said that before she had endometriosis, she ran every day. For the six months**

prior to her endometriosis surgery, "my level of exercise was severely reduced."

***

I became an expert at covering up my illness. I certainly knew that my husband did not want to be bothered or inconvenienced, and he made it sound like our friends felt the same way. The subject was also hard to discuss with friends – I mean, female menstrual issues? Who wants to talk about that? So, when friends were around, I smiled and laughed, even though I had a migraine. I smiled and laughed even through moderate cramps. I smiled and laughed while at the same time worrying if blood would seep onto my clothes or stain a chair. I smiled and laughed even though I secretly wondered what they would think if I left a thoroughly soaked maxi pad, wrapped up in half a roll of bathroom tissue, in their bathroom wastebasket. If I sneezed and felt a huge gush of blood come out of me, I continued to smile and laugh. A huge cramp would hit. "Oh, no," I thought. "Is a severe attack about to hit me?" But no, I would smile and laugh through it all. I held out as long as possible because I didn't want to be the "party pooper." I was more concerned about their feelings than my own. My husband had convinced me that they would all just sigh and nod their head in disapproval if I dare leave because of my pain. I now think I may have gotten much more support from them if they knew the truth, but I lived in fear – fear of rejection, fear of disgust, and fear of judgment for this thing that I had absolutely no control over.

2002

"Anyone can fake being sick, but it takes a really strong woman to fake being well."

-Jill Fuersich

In January, I saw my internist again for persistent nasal congestion and headaches. Her diagnosis? Sinusitis vs. chronic allergies. She prescribed Nasocort® nasal spray and Avelox®.

> ***Medication information***: **Nasocort®, also known as triamcinolone acetonide, is a corticosteroid nasal spray used to treat seasonal and year-round allergy symptoms. Avelox®, also known as moxifloxacin, is an antibiotic used to treat infections of the respiratory tract. It is also used to treat pelvic inflammatory disease.**

Finally, in April 2002, I had enough. My frustration turned into extreme outrage as I realized this behemoth inside me had negatively impacted my life for over 10 years. During the next follow-up visit with my gynecologist, I was adamant about doing further testing to see what was going on with me. She agreed to send me to have a transabdominal and transvaginal ultrasound to get a good look at what was going on inside my uterus. This transvaginal ultrasound was extremely painful. The tech who performed the exam had to push the probe far to each side to get a good look at my ovaries. I thought I was going to come off the table because it hurt so bad.

According to the radiologist's report, the uterus was levoverted as was previously reported. This means that it was leaning over toward one side of my abdomen (the left side in my case). That made sense to me because 99% of the pain that I felt was on the left side of my pelvis. Additionally, the radiologist stated the following:

"Endometrial lining: 5 mm in thickness but there is evidence for a possible 5 mm polyp along the left side of the fundal endometrium. Consider hysteroscopy or sonohysteroscopy."

Note: An endometrial or uterine polyp is a growth protruding from the uterine wall into the uterus. It is usually benign, but there have been cases where they become cancerous. It develops from overgrowth of the endometrium, and it is estrogen sensitive.

My gynecologist told me that this polyp was probably causing my symptoms as they can cause infertility, irregular or heavy periods, and bleeding between periods. I was skeptical. I had many ultrasounds in previous years, but this polyp was just found during this last ultrasound. Was this a new polyp, or had it always been there and was missed on all the other ultrasounds? I had become very cynical and questioned everything a doctor told me. I became my own advocate by doing my research and going to appointments armed with scientific facts. Some of the doctors seemed to take offense, but that did not matter to me. I just wanted an answer, and the doctors who I had seen could not give that to me.

My gynecologist ordered a sonohysterogram. She warned me that I might have some cramping during the procedure.

Note: A sonohysterogram is a minimally invasive procedure that is used to visualize and evaluate uterine abnormalities such as fibroids and polyps. This procedure is also used to evaluate women who suffer from infertility or repeat miscarriages. A transvaginal ultrasound is done first to locate abnormalities and examine the inside of the uterus. When this is done, the probe is removed, and a speculum is inserted. The cervix is cleansed, and a small catheter is placed into the uterus. Next, the speculum is removed, and the transvaginal

ultrasound probe is reinserted. Sterile saline is injected into the uterus through the catheter, and the ultrasound is performed. The entire procedure usually takes about 30 minutes to perform.

Although terrified, I agreed to the procedure. My Pap smears were painful, and the last transvaginal ultrasound that I had was particularly excruciating, so I could not even begin to think how painful this sonohysterogram would be. I was in a complete panic before the test. I asked my husband to go with me even though he wasn't the most supportive person. At least someone I knew would be there with me.

***

"I don't understand what we're doing. What do you want me to do?" I asked.

"I already told you," replied my husband.

"Well, I don't understand this financial stuff. Why can't you call?"

"Because your name is on the account."

Suddenly, I felt this overwhelming sense that walls were closing in around me. It felt like everyone was yelling at me:

"Call and get this done!"

"I want this case out today!"

"Try a gluten-free diet. That will help you."

"Try this doctor. He will help you."

"Exercise more!"

"Why are you always canceling plans?"

When are you going to have a baby?"

"I can't find anything wrong with you."

"All the tests are normal."

"STOP!" I exclaimed. "I am not dealing with this now!" I exclaimed as I stomped up the stairs to the bedroom.

"Where are you going??" my husband demanded.

I ignored him, went into the bedroom, sat on the edge of the bed, and ran my fingers through my hair. I was at a breaking point. I just needed some quiet time. I wanted to scream at everyone to shut the hell up and leave me alone. I stayed in the bedroom the rest of the night. Exasperated, I fell asleep without eating dinner.

***

I expected the sonohysterogram would be painful, but to my surprise, it was quite painless other than the usual discomfort from the speculum and probe. I watched the whole thing on a TV screen, and I could clearly see the polyp toward the top of my uterus. After the procedure, I got dressed, and my husband and I left. I was so relieved that the procedure wasn't nearly as painful as I had expected.

About 10-15 minutes later, as we waited in bumper-to-bumper traffic (it was rush hour in northern Virginia), I started to feel bloated. A few minutes later, severe cramps started. I was doubled over in the front passenger seat of the car.

"We have to get out of this traffic!" I exclaimed as another wave of pain hit me. I became nauseous and thought I was going to vomit.

My husband was desperately trying to move into the right-hand lane to exit off the road, but other drivers would not let him over.

"Get over!" I exclaimed.

"I'm trying!"

Doubled over and nauseated, I contemplated opening the door and vomiting in the middle of traffic. But instead, I just took some deep breaths. Sweat started to roll down the sides of my face.

I looked at the drivers in the right-hand lane. "Oh, come on!" I yelled. Finally, my husband was able to get over, and he took the next exit.

"Go to Wendy's," I said.

I got out of the car and went into the Wendy's bathroom where I had a huge bowel movement. Although I was still a little sick to my stomach, that bowel movement relieved enough of my symptoms that I thought I could make it home. I returned to the car.

"Better?" asked my husband.

"Not good, but better," I responded.

I reclined the seat, closed my eyes, and rested. What are the chances that a severe attack of IBS happens right after I had an invasive procedure involving my uterus? The cause of my pain was my uterus, and I knew it. Now, getting my doctors to agree with me would be another story.

> *Note:* **Years later after I learned about adenomyosis, I have an idea why my uterus was levoverted to the left. My ultrasound report said that my uterus was levoverted to the left. That is where I felt most of my pain - on the left side where the lower part of the bowel is located. Could it be that the uterus became irritated from the saline injected during the sonohysterogram? Or perhaps adhesions were present which played a role in this? I was not given any instruction to empty my bowel before the procedure, and I think may have helped to prevent this attack.**

By the time we arrived home, I was fine again.

After this happened, I returned to my internist. I told her that I had severe cramping pain after the sonohysterogram. I told her that this has to be somehow linked to my uterus; however, during her exam, she noted discomfort in my lower spine and gluteus muscle. In her notes, she wrote down:

"Muscle spasm vs. Uterine cramps vs. UTI"

Reallly? A urinary tract infection? I mean, really?

She put me on Cipro® and told me to use Bengay®. I found out later that the urine test came back negative which did not surprise me at all. I didn't need that test, but she insisted. She also ran a CBC, and the results came back as normal – no anemia and normal white blood cell counts.

> ***Medication facts*: Cipro® is a fluoroquinolone antibiotic that is used to treat bacterial infections such as sinus, bone, joint, lung, and skin infections. This antibiotic makes the patient more susceptible to the effects of the sun, so it is particularly important to protect against sunburn when using this medication. Bengay® is an analgesic heat rub used to treat pain from sore muscles, arthritis, bruises, etc. The active ingredients in this product are methyl salicylate, menthol, and camphor.**

***

The following is an excerpt from the radiologist's report regarding my sonohysterogram:

> *"The preliminary transabdominal study shows the uterus to be normal for size measuring 7.4 cm for length. No adnexal abnormality is seen. No free fluid in the pelvis. Following prepping of the cervix, a 5 French catheter was introduced through the cervical os and a small*

amount of sterile saline was injected during ultrasound observation. A broad based pedunculated endometrial polyp is seen at the level of the uterine midbody just to the left of midline with a maximum diameter of 7 mm. The polyp is estimated to be approximately 4 cm from the level of the cervix. The endometrium is otherwise thin and uniform with single wall thickness of 1-2 mm."

At some point during this time, I was switched to yet another birth control pill. This time, my gynecologist wanted me to try continuous Lo Estrin®. I stayed on this pill for the next several years.

***

The next step was to schedule a hysteroscopy for removal of the endometrial polyp. This surgery was scheduled for October 2002.

Both my husband and my mom were there for me during my hysteroscopy. While in the waiting room, my mom and my husband had a conversation about my situation.

"I sure hope this surgery will finally give her some relief," she said.

"Me too," he responded.

"She's been through so much."

"Yeah. I just need to keep her working," said my husband.

My mom didn't respond, but she thought that was a strange comment to make at that time. She told me about that comment years later and how it made her feel. I told her that it didn't surprise me one bit as all he seemed to be concerned with during our marriage was making money, playing poker, and playing golf. He didn't seem to be overly concerned for me or my chronic health problem.

During this surgery, it was noted that I had cervical stenosis and a septate bicornuate uterus.

> ***Note:*** **Cervical stenosis refers to the narrowing of the passage through the cervix. It can be congenital or acquired. Acquired cases of cervical stenosis may be caused by cervical surgery, endometrial ablation, radiation treatment, or uterine cancer. This condition is usually not symptomatic and normally does not require treatment. If symptoms are present, they can include the following:**
>
> - **Amenorrhea**
> - **Dysmenorrhea**
> - **Infertility**
> - **Pooling of blood in the body of the uterus which can lead to a backward flow. This can result in the development of endometriosis.**
>
> **If symptoms are problematic, treatment may be done to improve the condition. Cervical dilation and/or placement of a cervical stent may help.**
>
> **A bicornuate uterus is also known as a "heart-shaped" uterus. This type of uterus has two "horns" which occurs because of a congenital abnormality of the fusion of the Müllerian ducts during fetal development. Problems include cervical incompetence, miscarriage, pre-term births, breech births, retained placenta, and birth defects.**

My gynecologist spoke to me after the surgery and told me that everything went fine. The polyp had been removed. However, I remember a comment that she made that bothered me. She mentioned that she was able to view the right side of the uterus, but the left side was very dark, and she didn't feel comfortable going too deep for fear that she would puncture the uterine wall. My heart sunk when she told me that. Most of my pain was on the left side, and that is the side of the uterus that needed to be viewed to determine the cause of my pain. I was not convinced at that point that the surgery would be successful.

The following is an excerpt from the operative report from my hysteroscopy:

"The cervix was grasped with a tooth tenaculum, and an attempt was made to sound the uterus. The uterine sound was unable to be passed through the cervix. A tonsil hemostat was then used to attempt to dilate the cervix. This was unsuccessful. Then, an os finder was used to successfully dilate the cervix. The uterus sounded to 8 cm. Using Pratt graduated dilators, the cervix was dilated sufficiently to admit the 0-degree hysteroscope. The hysteroscope was inserted using glycine as the distention medium. The endocervix appeared normal. Just inside the level of the internal os, there was a polyp noted that had a smooth, pale surface. It was linear and may have even represented a small fibroid. The hysteroscope was advanced further, and it was noted that the uterus had a slightly septate bicornuate appearance. The right horn was rather shallow. The left horn was deeper. The endometrium itself appeared pale and unremarkable. The right ostia was visualized. The left ostium was difficult to visualize; however, the left horn appeared somewhat narrow and was difficult to be certain whether the ostium was identified. The hysteroscope was removed. The Corson polyp forceps were introduced yielding a 1 cm x 7 cm, firm, polypoid mass consistent with either polyp or small fibroid. The small uterine curet was then used to curet the endometrial surface yielding moderate tissue. The hysteroscope was then reintroduced showing the resolution of the polypoid mass and freshly curetted endometrium."

The pathology report from this surgery stated the following:

> *"Endometrial polyp, fragments of endometrium showing atrophic glands with mild decidual change of stroma consistent with hormone effect."*

> ***Note***: **Atrophic glands refer to cuboidal and/or columnar epithelium that have little to no chromosome activity. These types of glands are usually seen in prepubertal girls or post-menopausal women but can also be seen in women who are perimenopausal. These types of glands are usually a result of progesterone activity. They have also been noted in polyps.**

After surgery, there were no complications. I recovered for a few days at home and then resumed my normal activities.

***

During my post op visit, my gynecologist explained that the dysfunctional uterine bleeding that I had been experiencing was probably a result of the polyp that was present in my uterus. She believed that removal of this polyp would resolve a lot of the symptoms that I had experienced. I must admit I was pessimistic. How many times have I heard that "this surgery should resolve your pain"? Yet the pain always returned. It was extraordinarily difficult to be optimistic.

This was the last time I saw this gynecologist. My husband and I were getting ready to move to San Antonio, Texas. At this point, I was somewhat stable on continuous birth control (Lo Estrin®) and Sarafem® for PMDD.

My pain did return within a few months. My husband asked me what I was going to do.

"Nothing," I replied. He just looked at me.

"Nothing," I reiterated. "I am getting nowhere. All I am doing is using up all my sick time to sit in a damn doctor's office to hear the same damn thing repeatedly. Let's face it – they can't help me, and I am sick of wasting my time."

He didn't respond.

Texas (2003-2007)

2003

*"Fatigue is a very common symptom with [adenomyosis],
since lower blood counts, also known as 'anemia,' can
prevent patients from performing normal activities, and
often exercise is limited."*

Dr. Natalya Danilyants

I left the Washington D.C. area on a continuous birth control pill
(Lo Estrin®) which would cause me to have only four menstrual
periods per year. I was still taking Sarafem® for depression, and I
just had an endometrial polyp removed from my uterus. Even
though things were a bit better, I still believed that the root cause
of my issues had not yet been addressed.

My symptoms remained under control for several years. I didn't
want to change what had been prescribed for fear that all the
problems would return full force. I just stayed with the program
as it was when I left northern Virginia. However, things started
to go downhill in 2006.

I started to have some bad attacks of abdominal pain with severe
stomach bloating that would just hit me unexpectedly. One
morning as I was got ready to go to work, my stomach suddenly
bloated up to the size of about a 4-month pregnancy again. A
few minutes later, I was doubled over in severe pain. In the
middle of this, I somehow managed to get to the phone and call
into work, telling them that I would be there when I felt better.

***

My husband and I went to Virginia during Christmas. I was not
on my period at the time, so I expected this trip to go well and
with little if any pain. The first night we were there, I woke up at
about 3 a.m. completely soaked in sweat. I was stunned at how
wet I was – my hair line was completely wet, the neckline and
back of my shirt was damp, and I was sweating profusely

underneath my breasts. I got up and walked out into the hallway as to not disturb my husband. I moved my shirt back and forth to cool off, and then I went to the bathroom. Beads of sweat covered my face. I rinsed my face with chilly water and dried it off, and then waved my hand in front of my face to help myself cool off some more. I moved my shirt back and forth for several minutes until I finally cooled off enough that I could return to bed. While lying in bed, I stared at the ceiling and wondered if this was the beginning of menopause or if this was somehow related to my health problems. The next morning, I told my mom and husband what happened.

"I had something really weird happen to me in the middle of the night last night."

"What happened?" asked my mom.

"I think I had a hot flash. I woke up soaked in sweat, and I had to get up and cool myself off for about ten minutes before it finally let up."

My mom looked at me inquisitively. "That's odd."

"I know. I don't know if it's the beginning of menopause or if this is somehow related to all the other stuff that's been happening to me."

"Did you have pain?" she asked.

"No. No pain. Just profuse sweating."

"I didn't have much of an issue with hot flashes during menopause, so I can't help much. But I did hear someone describe it once. She said it was like heat moving throughout your body and then going out the top of your head," my mom said as she laughed.

"Really?" I said as I laughed with her.

"Yeah, I'm not kidding. That's what I heard!"

"Well, it wasn't like that last night. I just woke up sweating, hot all over. I guess that could have been some kind of hormone fluctuation."

"Maybe," she responded.

***

The continuous birth control therapy helped me because I was only having four periods a year. However, when the periods did come, they were exceptionally long, sometimes lasting a full two weeks. The bleeding was horrendously heavy, and I would have terrible cramping along with PMDD. The fatigue and headaches were debilitating, and there were many days I would come home from work and go straight to bed without even eating dinner. It took every ounce of energy I had to get through my workday. I was also passing blood clots as large as the palm of my hand and was also dizzy and lightheaded, probably due to the amount of blood lost. In addition to all of this, I had spotting for several days once the heavy bleeding stopped, and I never knew exactly when the spotting would stop. It never failed – I would think the spotting had stopped, and I would stop wearing panty liners. Later, when I went to the bathroom, the spotting would have started again. I ruined numerous pairs of underwear because of this and was annoyed beyond belief.

2004

"Headaches in women, especially migraines, are related to changes in the levels of estrogen. Levels of estrogen drop immediately before the start of your menstrual flow (menses)."

-Cleveland Clinic

I began to work at a cytogenetics lab at the University of Texas. One day while working in the lab, I started to develop another menstrual migraine. I was bleeding extremely heavily, and I knew this headache was destined to become severe. However, I only had about 1 ½ hours left to work, so I decided to just push through.

I was so relieved when it was time to leave.

New employees at the university had to park off campus. Every day, I had to wait for a bus to take me to the parking lot where my car was located. I walked out to the bus stop and waited for the bus which came about 10 minutes later.

I sat down on the bus next to a window. I laid my head against the window and closed my eyes.

"I hope we get to the parking lot soon, "I thought to myself. "My head is about to explode." I also realized that I needed to change my maxi pad, but that would have to wait until I got home.

The bus did not go directly to my parking lot. Instead, it made two trips around campus. By the time the driver was finished with his second trip, the bus was packed, and it was very loud. The noise made me nauseous, and I was miserable. I wanted so bad to get off and just walk to my car.

The bus finally arrived at my parking lot. I slowly walked to my car as my head pounded. My eyes hurt. I felt like I could barely hold them open, and I still had a 30-minute drive home.

At each stop light, I closed my eyes for a few seconds at a time. I could have very easily fallen asleep, but I remembered my experience in Virginia, and I made sure to open my eyes every few seconds or so.

Last year, I authored a book called *Adenomyosis: The Women Speak*. This book included surveys of women from the Adenomyosis Fighter's Support Group on Facebook. One of the questions asked was about fatigue levels, and one of the women stated that she had fallen asleep at a stop light. I could not believe it! I totally understood that, and even though I never did fall asleep at a stoplight, I certainly came close to doing so!

***

One morning, I woke up to severe right-sided pain. This pain was a bit different since most of the time, my pain was left-sided. It was unrelenting, sharp pain. I asked my husband to take me to the ER again, and he reluctantly did so. We barely talked on our way there.

In the ER, I once again explained all my symptoms to the nurse.

"They are going to want to do a pelvic," said the nurse.

"Here we go again," I thought to myself. "Same old, same old…"

The nurse took me to another room where I undressed. She put me in stirrups, but these stirrups were not like the ones I was used to. These must have been special childbirth stirrups. My feet were high up in the air, and my butt was open for all the world to see. It was such an uncomfortable position, and I could not wait for the exam to be over.

The ER doctor came in. I had not seen him before, and here I was in this horribly vulnerable position.

"Sounds like an ovarian cyst," he said to me without asking me about my symptoms at all. He got all his information from the

180

nurse and my chart, and he had already diagnosed me without even meeting me.

He immediately started the exam, and even though I was in pain, he pushed my legs wide open.

"Open up your legs!" he exclaimed as he pushed my legs out farther.

I was in an extremely vulnerable position, in pain, and now this doctor is yelling at me and pushing my legs wide open.

"Relax!" he said forcefully.

"Right. I am going to relax while you are yelling at me? Seriously?" I thought to myself.

He performed the exam but complained the entire time that I needed to relax and open my legs. It was the most painful pelvic exam of my life. I was furious by the time it was over.

He shook his head, clearly annoyed, and said, "It's probably an ovarian cyst. I'll give you some pain relievers."

That was it. A horrible pelvic exam. A guess as to what it was. No confirmatory test such as an ultrasound. Treatment was to take a pain reliever. Well, that was a couple of wasted hours of my life that I cannot get back.

Looking back on that exam, I should have just gotten out of the stirrups and left. I also should have reported him for his disgusting bed-side manner. However, at the time, I was laser-focused on controlling my symptoms. I did not have the time or energy to fight that battle too.

***

"When are you all going to have a child?" my mother-in-law asked yet again. I was 39 years old, so I think she was really concerned at this point that she wasn't going to have any more grandchildren.

"We have been trying, but I am having all of these medical problems," I said angrily, disgusted that this conversation even started.

"The two of you would be the perfect parents," she said. "It would just be so wrong for the two of you to have no children."

"Yes, I know, but..."

"No, listen to me, Maria. You need to have children. You are really going to regret it if you don't. Who is going to take care of you when you get older?"

My heart ached. I already knew this. It already hurt every single day knowing that I probably would never have any children. I knew that I may grow old alone. That thought hurt me every single day, and what she just said to me just added more agony on top of the hurt I already felt.

"Listen, we have tried for years," I retorted.

"But..."

"No, you aren't listening," I said. "We have tried. It's not like I don't want children. I do!"

"Well, then get to it!" she responded.

I sighed, turned around, and left.

2005

"I'm so tired of seeing on my social media, 'Why don't you have kids? Why don't you have kids?' You don't know what I'm going through, you have no idea. It is really difficult. I have had some not-so-happy, traumatic moments."

-Tyra Banks

"I want a son," my husband said as we drove home.

"What?" I asked.

"I want a son."

I looked out the window and hesitated for a minute. I was stunned at his statement since I thought we had come to understand that we probably would never be able to have our own child.

"Well, I can come off birth control again and we can try again if you want to."

He was silent.

"Well?"

"Yeah," he responded. "Yeah, I really want a son."

I hesitated again. "OK, we'll try again then."

It was a bit of a stressed discussion because I think deep down inside, we both knew that the chances of a pregnancy were slim to none. I was 39 years old with a long history of menstrual issues and infertility. I realized that he still did not understand anything about my health problems even after all these years. He still did not realize the amount of pain I had endured over the years, and he still did not understand the emotional toll it had taken on me, having to go through all the pain, exams, and medication side effects. But even after going through all of that, I still was willing to go through more pain to become pregnant. I came off birth control while we tried again for a pregnancy.

One night as we sat in our living room watching television, my stomach began to bloat. I had only told my husband about the bloating – he had never paid close attention to the bloating mostly because at its worst, I was alone in the bathroom in severe pain. This time, however, the pain did not start immediately. I just sat there, hoping that the pain would never start. As I rubbed my enlarged stomach, I looked over at my husband.

"Hey," I said. "You have never seen me really bloated. Look at my stomach."

He glanced over as I held my shirt up so he could see it. His eyes widened.

"What is wrong with you?" he said.

"I told you! This is what it is like. This is how I bloat!"

He shook his head and looked back at the television. "You need to see a doctor about that."

"What do you think I've been doing??" I demanded.

I could not believe he said that. He clearly was clueless about this disease. I was invisible to him, and I knew at this point that my misery would never be visible to him because he did not want it to be. Maybe it was denial, lack of compassion, or plain ignorance, but whatever it was, he would never understand. I felt like my heart broke in two.

***

During an annual physical, some bloodwork that was done showed that my cholesterol was elevated. My general practitioner suggested that I go on Crestor®. I did start this statin drug, and my cholesterol levels decreased quite dramatically. I didn't think much else about this – I just assumed I was getting older, and this was just part of life.

> ***Medication facts***: **Crestor® is a type of statin drug used to lower bad cholesterol, slow progression of atherosclerosis, and reduce the risk of heart attack. Side effects include weakness, abdominal pain, headache, nausea, and muscle aches. There is also a risk of kidney and/or liver damage. Specifically, it can cause rhabdomyolysis which is a severe form of muscle damage that can lead to severe kidney problems and even death.**

***

I turned 40 in 2005, so my husband surprised me with a cruise to Alaska. I was so excited to go, but in the back of my mind, I wondered if I would enjoy this trip. Would this pain rear its ugly head again?

Everything was going so well, and then on the second night, I woke up to that all familiar cramping pain again. I couldn't believe it! I walked to the bathroom, doubled over, and I tried to go to the bathroom. I was able to urinate, but again, I couldn't have a bowel movement. I started to panic.

This time, I sat on the end of the bed as my husband slept. I closed my eyes and breathed deeply to calm myself down, but the cramps continued. I stood up to go to the bathroom, and I felt like I was going to pass out. I slowly walked doubled over to the bathroom while holding onto the walls and sink. I tried once again to have a bowel movement, but again, nothing happened. I returned to the bed and continued the deep breathing. After a few minutes, I noticed that the pain had slowly improved, so I decided to get back in bed, hoping that this reduction in pain was a good sign. I was able to fall back to sleep.

In the morning, I felt fine. I don't know why this attack suddenly stopped without the necessity of having a bowel movement, but I sure was happy that it did stop. I forgot all about it and continued to enjoy my all-time favorite vacation. Alaska was beautiful!

***

Since I was 40 years old, a mammogram was recommended when I had my annual physical. I remembered my first experience, and I was a bit nervous, but I agreed to one since there is a history of breast cancer in my family.

I was taken back, and we went through the same procedure as before. Not much had changed over the years as far as I could tell, but I was told that the machines were much more sensitive, so that made me feel good. If something were there, they would be more likely to find it as compared to the one I had about 15 years earlier.

After the mammogram, I was told to wait in a small room. The tech said the radiologist was going to look at the films and they would let me know if they needed more pictures. This was new. Last time, I was sent home after the mammogram. This was a bit nerve-racking, but I just sat there and looked at a magazine. About 15 minutes later, the nurse came back in.

"We need to take more pictures," she said. "Come with me."

I stood up and followed her as my heart beat out of my chest.

"Did the radiologist see something?" I asked.

"Well, you have very dense breast tissue. There are a few spots that he wants to take a second look at just to be sure."

The nurse looked at me, and I am sure she saw that I was worried.

"Don't worry," she said as we walked into the room with the mammogram machine. "This happens quite often, and almost always, it's nothing."

That made me feel a bit better, but with my family history, I just could not shake that feeling of dread. The new pictures that she took were quite painful as she really had to push the two plates down hard to flatten my breast. I groaned as she did this.

"I know this hurts," she said. "It will take just a few seconds. Hang in there."

"OK," I whispered as I tried to breathe through the discomfort.

Before I knew it, it was over. She brought me back to the waiting room where I had to wait once again. Was it going to be good news? Did I have breast cancer?

Instead of reading the magazine, I just sat there, picking at my fingernails. I was so frightened. Chemotherapy? Radiation? What would my husband think?

Finally, that door opened. "You're good to go," she said.

"Everything is OK?" I asked.

"Yep. Everything looks good. You just have fibrocystic disease, but no cancer."

"Oh, thank God," I said as I breathed a sigh of relief.

2006

"Social traditions can inaccurately teach women from a young age that heavy bleeding and pain during periods are normal, but these symptoms if left untreated can intensify over time, leading to lower quality of life, pain during sexual intercourse, and issues with fertility."

-Dr. Kimberly A. Cho

All of the symptoms worsened as I aged. The bleeding became more prolonged, and the spotting seemed endless. The large clots became more numerous. The pain worsened even though I was taking fish oil and eating lots of salads. My age made it harder and harder for me to tolerate the pain and heavy bleeding. I just did not have the stamina for it anymore. We finally gave up our efforts for a pregnancy, and I went back on birth control.

After being on continuous birth control for three months, I stopped taking them for a week for my breakthrough bleed that happened four times a year. On the third day, I woke up to heavy bleeding. After eating breakfast, I started to have severe bowel cramping. As I sat on the steps outside of my bathroom trying to breathe through the cramps, my husband walked by.

"It's happening again," I said as I clutched my pelvis.

A cramp hit me full force, and I stood up, doubled over, and tried to walk to the bathroom.

"Are you going to work?"

I didn't have enough energy to get angry at him at that moment. "No," I responded and shut the bathroom door.

Once the cramps let up, I laid in bed and thought about what he had said to me. It had been sixteen years of this nightmare, and he still didn't get it. All he cared about was that I kept my job and continued to work. That's it. I realized that he didn't mean "in sickness and in health." He wanted a healthy wife. I knew at that point that he did not care one bit about what I had gone through, and it made me sad, frustrated, and angry. I did not have the emotional and mental support that I so desperately needed through this nightmare journey.

2007

"Hysterectomy is a cure when adenomyosis is the only cause for painful periods...Hysterectomy is not a cure for endometriosis, as endometriosis exists outside the uterus. Hysterectomy is a treatment option for endometriosis and will only be successful if the endometriosis is completely removed from every area."

-Dr. Tamer Seckin

Finally, in 2007, I found a great gynecologist in San Antonio. She had the best bed-side manner, and she took as much time as I needed to explain everything that I had been through over the seventeen previous years. We thoroughly went through all my symptoms, and although she could not diagnose me at that point, she did offer something that sounded promising at the time.

"There is a procedure called an endometrial ablation. This burns off the endometrial lining of the uterus so that you either will not bleed or will have only minimal bleeding during the time that you are supposed to have your period. The drawback to this procedure, however, is that pregnancy is not advised after this procedure is done. That means that you won't be able to have any children."

"Oh, I could care less about that at this point," I replied. "I am just so sick of dealing with this."

"What about your husband? Would he be OK with this?"

"Oh, I am sure he would be OK with it. We've given up on kids."

"Well, why don't you go home and talk to him about it. Think about it and let me know. Here's a pamphlet on it."

She handed me the pamphlet on the NovaSure® ablation. I thanked her, went home, read it, and talked to my husband just as she asked me to do. However, I had already made my mind up. I was having this surgery whether my husband approved or not.

> *Note:* **An endometrial ablation is a medical procedure that destroys the endometrial layer inside the uterus. This procedure is typically done on women who are suffering from excessive blood loss during menstruation that is not controlled by medication. An endometrial ablation is generally not recommended for women with adenomyosis, especially in women with deep adenomyosis. According to the Sydney Fibroid Clinic in Sydney Australia, "...studies have shown the presence of adenomyosis predicts a poor outcome [of an endometrial ablation] and usually results in persistent or worsening period pain."**
>
> **Endometrial ablation is discussed at length later in this book.**

***

I was hopeful but also nervous on the morning of the ablation. Would this finally be the answer to all these problems? Would I wake up in pain? How long will it take for me to fully recover? I usually had very few issues with my other surgeries, but you never really know for sure how you are going to respond to a surgical procedure.

I woke up after the ablation with exceptionally light cramping. It was one of the easier surgeries that I had since this whole thing began. I was given some pain medication, but the pain was short-lived. By the time I got home, I really did not have any pain, and I spent the rest of the day sleeping.

The next morning, I got up and went to the bathroom. No bleeding! Maybe this worked?!? Oh, I sure hoped so.

A few hours later, I went to the bathroom again. This time there was blood. It was not a lot of blood, but it was there. My heart sunk, but I did not panic because I just had surgery. Maybe this was normal. I just had to be patient.

By the next morning, I realized that this ablation didn't work. I was bleeding quite a bit, so my husband took me to the emergency room. After explaining my situation, the ER doctor performed a pelvic exam. She was much gentler than that other doctor who was so rough, but even so, this was the most painful pelvic I had ever had. It felt like she was tearing my vagina in two when she inserted the speculum.

"Owww!!" I screeched as she inserted the speculum.

She quickly removed it as I broke down in tears.

"Get a smaller one," the doctor said to the nurse.

The nurse came back with a smaller speculum. "I'm going to try again," she said.

She inserted it as I cried. I turned to my husband.

"It really hurts," I said.

"It's almost over," said my husband.

"Hang in there," said the doctor.

The tearing and burning sensations were horrendous. Tears trickled down my face, and I just counted the seconds until that speculum was removed. When it was over and she removed the speculum, I was so relieved!

She noted the bleeding but could not give me a reason as to why it was happening. She suggested that I make an appointment to see my gynecologist, so that is what I did. I felt totally defeated.

***

At the appointment, my gynecologist examined me again, and it was painful.

No!!" I exclaimed as I started to cry again.

She quickly removed the speculum.

"It hurts like it did in the ER," I said through the tears.

"OK," she said.

We waited a minute, and then she tried to examine me again very gently.

"Are you doing OK?"

"I just want it to be over," I said as I wiped the tears from my face.

 A worried look came over her face.

"Oh, this is too much bleeding," she said. "This isn't normal."

"So, what now?"

"You can sit up," she said as she helped me up.

"Well, I am not sure. I have done so many of these ablations, and I have never seen bleeding like this after any of them."

I looked straight into her eyes. "Can I have a hysterectomy?"

She looked into my eyes. "Yes," she said. "I think that's a good idea. Since the ablation didn't work, that would be our next step."

"I'm ready. I just don't want to do this anymore."

"I completely understand," she said. She wrote some notes in my chart. "Go ahead and get dressed, and the ladies at the front desk will help you to schedule surgery."

"Thank you so much," I replied as she moved toward the door.

"Of course," she replied.

***

Several months later, I was at the hospital getting ready to have a hysterectomy. We had agreed that removal of the uterus was all that was necessary – I would keep my ovaries and cervix. She told me that if she took the ovaries, I would immediately go into premature menopause, and she did not recommend that. The hysterectomy was going to be a laparoscopic supracervical hysterectomy. She explained to me that with this kind of hysterectomy, there is a possibility that she would not be able to get all the uterine tissue removed during surgery. This meant that I may continue to have light spotting during the time of menstruation after the surgery and until menopause.

> *Note*: **A laparoscopic supracervical hysterectomy is a minimally invasive procedure in which only the uterus is removed. The cervix is left in place.**
> **Sometimes the fallopian tubes are removed if they are diseased or if there is another reason to remove them. Each case is different. Please refer to the Hysterectomy section later in this book for more information.**

The surgery went very well. I did not have any complications. My mom came to Texas to be with me during this time, and her support was a tremendous comfort to me. I was up and walking around the day after surgery, and she could not believe that I came out of it as easily as I did. The morning after surgery, I had one small bout of abdominal pain that lasted about fifteen minutes, but it resolved quickly after I had a bowel movement.

A few days later, we had a post op appointment with my gynecologist. Little did I know that this appointment would finally answer that question that plagued me for seventeen years.

My mom and I sat patiently in the room as we waited for the gynecologist. She finally came in, sat down, and looked at me.

"How are you feeling?"

"I actually feel good. I came through the surgery without any issues, and I have no pain or bleeding right now."

"Great!" she exclaimed. "Happy to hear that."

She looked down at my chart.

"Well, I have the pathology results from your hysterectomy. It turns out that you had a condition called adenomyosis. This is where the endometrium invades the uterine muscle. We do not know why it happens, but it can cause heavy bleeding and severe pain. There were also multiple possible fibroids found throughout the uterine wall."

I felt like the weight of the world had been lifted off my shoulders. Finally, I had an answer. Finally, I can prove to people around me that I was not faking anything. Finally, I can go out in public without fear of another attack. Finally, I can have some peace and enjoy life.

That evening, I broke the news to my husband as he arrived home from work.

"I finally got an answer," I said with a smile. My mom sat next to me on the couch as we shared the news that they found adenomyosis. My husband listened but did not really react.

"Well, it's good that we finally have an answer," he said.

"Finally," I said.

My mom and I continued to talk while my husband went upstairs to change his clothes. He was gone for a while, but we were too involved in our conversation to notice. When he came back, he walked into the living room with tears in his eyes. He sat down next to me.

"I just looked up adenomyosis online," he said. "I didn't realize that you were going through all that." He hugged me, and I felt a combination of relief and confusion. I did not know what to think at that moment. The three of us talked a little bit more about what I went through, and then my husband left to pick up dinner. When he walked out, I looked at my mom.

"That was a little strange," I said.

"I think he finally gets it," replied my mom.

"I am not so sure," I said. "Why didn't he believe me all these years? Why did it take a pathologist saying I had adenomyosis before he finally believed that I had a problem?"

"Well, I think he realizes now that he was wrong."

"Hmmm," I responded. I felt his reaction was not genuine. It was just a gut feeling, but I just did not believe that he was being authentic. To be honest, I thought he was doing it for show in front of my mom. It just did not sit right with me.

The next day, I sent roses to my gynecologist. I wanted her to know how much it meant to me that she was finally able to accurately diagnose my condition. She will never know how she impacted my life – she literally gave me my life back!

> ***Note***: **Moradi et al. (2014) stated that when women finally received their correct diagnosis, they felt relieved. They were glad to know that it wasn't all in their head. That is exactly how I felt after my diagnosis of adenomyosis.**

The Post-Hysterectomy Years

"We all understood that there was no way I was going to achieve the things I wanted to achieve or was meant to achieve if that hysterectomy didn't happen. And I hope that for so many women, with an early enough diagnosis, they never even have to ask themselves that question."

Lena Durham

I did have spotting from the cervical stump for about seven years after my hysterectomy. It was annoying at best. The pain was completely gone, but I had to deal with this annoying spotting which was many times mixed with mucus, and it was disgusting. If I had to do it all over again, I would have had my cervix removed, but at the time, I wasn't educated very well about this type of hysterectomy. I hope this information will help others make the best choice for them. The bleeding finally stopped completely in 2014.

Since that time, I have never had a recurrence of an attack of severe abdominal pain. It has been fifteen years since my hysterectomy. In the end, this pain was not caused by IBS. All the procedures and medications used for the treatment of IBS were worthless in my case. This was entirely a problem with my uterus – a little known condition called adenomyosis.

Although I finally got relief from the abdominal pain that had caused all this suffering, other health problems continued to bother me, and even new things started to show up.

***

My allergy situation, which had been somewhat under control for years, started to worsen. I had finished the allergy shots, but I was slowly starting to have increased sinus trouble with each passing year. I was still curious as to why these symptoms seemed to flare during PMS prior to my hysterectomy. My head would be so congested during that time, and I constantly blew my nose and had fairly severe sinus headaches. Once menstrual spotting started, my sinus congestion would clear up until the next month. I thought this was strange, and I just could not imagine at all that sinus congestion could somehow be linked to female hormone fluctuations. I could not have been more surprised when I found out that this symptom could be linked to estrogen dominance. For more information, see sections on Estrogen Dominance and Allergies later in this book.

***

During the next few years, I enjoyed life much more as I no longer had to deal with severe abdominal pain and heavy bleeding. However, this was also the time that the public was starting to become aware of v and its importance in health. My general practitioner started to add a vitamin D test to my routine bloodwork, and it was found to be low on several occasions. After each test, I was given a prescription of vitamin D which was 50,000 IU once a week for 3 months. After each course, I was tested again, and my vitamin D levels were in the normal range. However, eventually it would revert back into the low range, and my next test was inevitably low again.

Just as I got used to feeling good, yet another health issue hit me unexpectedly. In the spring of 2009, as I was getting out of bed one morning, my right leg suddenly gave out from underneath me. I found out that I had a herniated disc in my lower back at L5/S1, and I needed to have a spinal fusion. In September of that same year, I had the fusion and was told after the surgery that one of the vertebrae in my lower back was broken. I had hoped that this surgery would fix the problem. Sadly, it did not. The bones failed to fuse, so I had a second fusion in 2010. The second surgery also failed. For some reason that could not be identified at the time, the bones in my lower back failed to fuse. I did not have any risk factors that we knew of for fusion failure.

However, the fact that I had persistently low vitamin D levels bothered me. Was this playing a factor in my failed fusions?

Before being taken back for my second surgery, I was given the antibiotic Ancef®. It was given to me as a drip through my IV. About 30 minutes or so after the drip was started, I turned bright red. My husband rushed out to get a nurse, and when the nurse saw me, she immediately stopped the drip. It turns out that I am allergic to this antibiotic. So, at that time, I could not take penicillin, sulfa (discovered allergy to sulfa in my teenage years) or Ancef® antibiotics due to allergy.

After the second failed spinal fusion, I decided to get a second opinion. The new doctor recommended that I go to another orthopedic surgeon who was an expert in complex spinal cases. I saw this new surgeon, and he recommended the following to try and determine why the bones in my back were not fusing properly.

1. *Assess vitamin D status since there is a history of low vitamin D levels.*
2. *Have a CT myelogram in order to get top quality images of my back prior to surgery.*
3. *Have an EMG done to evaluate my chronic radiculopathy (pain that spreads down my legs).*

During our discussion, I mentioned to the orthopedic surgeon that I had been on Crestor® for many years for high cholesterol. We decided to discontinue this medication since there was some concern that this drug may interfere with bone health.

> ***Note*: At that time, there was some concern about the effect of Crestor® on bone health. Today, many studies have found that Crestor® may, in fact, improve bone health. Specifically, a study by Chamani et al. (2021) showed that Crestor® increases expression of bone morphogenic protein-2 (BMP-2), glucocorticoids, TGF-β, ALP (alkaline phosphatase),**

type 1 collagen, and collagenase-1. Additionally, several studies have shown that statins may be effective against endometriosis as it has been shown to reduce the size of endometrial implants. One study in particular showed that the higher the dose of the statin, the more the endometrial implants regressed. However, another study showed that low doses of statins resulted in a low rate of osteoporosis while high doses of statins resulted in high rates of osteoporosis. This study concluded that the effect on bone health may be dose dependent (Leutner et al., 2019). Is it worth it to use high dose statins to treat endometriosis while risking bone health later in life? The details of this topic are beyond the scope of this book, but it is worth the time to perform more research on the effects of statins in adenomyosis and endometriosis.

I had all three tests done. The EMG was abnormal, but we decided that surgery may be able to help me. My vitamin D level was low again, so I was put on prescription strength vitamin D for 3 months prior to my third surgery. The CT myelogram required a head CT prior to the test, so I had that done; however, they found an aneurysm in my brain. The aneurysm took priority, so I had a coil and stent placed followed by a 3-month course of the blood thinner Plavix®. Once I was cleared, I was scheduled for my third back surgery.

***

While I waited to be cleared for my third spinal fusion, my in-laws, husband and I went to Las Vegas for vacation. When my mother-in-law saw me in the airport, she gave me a very cold "hello." I clearly could tell that she didn't want to have much to do with me. During that vacation, I felt like I didn't belong.

On the day we were leaving to go home, I waited by the door to the Luxor hotel for my husband who was checking out. I also was waiting for my in-laws who were still finishing up in their room. No one came for quite a while, so I started to look around. Through the hotel door, I saw my in-laws who were already outside. They had to have walked right past me, so I wondered why they didn't say anything to me. I walked outside and sat with them; however, I felt like a certain amount of tension. We went to the airport where we helped my in-laws find the gate where their plane was located. We decided to do this and then walk over to where our plane would take off. While my husband when to the counter to talk to the gate agent, my in-laws decided to stop by the bathroom. I took a seat at the gate while I waited on all of them. I pulled out my notebook and started to write (working on a past adenomyosis book) when I started to wonder where everyone was since it had been a while since we all parted ways. I turned around and scanned the area when I saw them. They all sat in an area away from me. Confused and feeling completely left out, I slowly packed up my stuff and went to sit with them.

"Why didn't they come and sit with me?" I wondered.

I asked my husband about this later, and he said there were no seats available around me. I thought for a moment, and I was even more confused. I knew there were open seats around me.

I was puzzled as I looked at him. I decided not to say anything else because I did not want to argue. But thoughts raced through my head.

"Why didn't he come and get me? Why is everyone being so stand offish?"

The whole thing was strange. I was getting some weird vibes, and I just could not make sense of it.

Looking back on this now, I realize that this kind of behavior toward me started after my hysterectomy. I feel like my mother-in-law's attitude changed toward me after my surgery because I would no longer be able to give her any more grandchildren.

There was absolutely nothing I could have done to change the fact that I could not have children.

Things started to make a little more sense after that vacation. Only two months later, my husband asked me for a divorce. Our divorce was finalized in 2014.

***

I had a third spinal fusion in 2012. Before the surgery, they put me on the antibiotic clindamycin. I was put to sleep, but when I woke up after surgery, I had an allergy tag on my wrist. When I asked the nurse why this tag was on my arm, she explained that just prior to the start of surgery, my heart rate dropped dangerously low, and they determined that I had an allergic reaction to clindamycin. I could not believe it! Now I was allergic to four antibiotics? I was stunned.

This time, in addition to using the routine hardware (rods and screws), bone morphogenic protein and bone marrow that was aspirated from my hip were used to aid in fusion. In addition, the fusion now involved L5/S2 (had to go down a level since S1 was no longer useful due to the previous two fusions). With all the extra effort put into the third surgery, it did succeed, and the bones finally fused although pain persists to this day.

> ***What we know today:*** **Progesterone is known to play a vital role in bone health. This fact intrigued me as I researched this topic because we know that estrogen dominance plays a role in adenomyosis and endometriosis. Could a problem with low progesterone levels play a role in my failed fusions? Well, it turns out that progesterone resistance is now known to be an issue in these disorders. More information on this topic can be found later in this book.**

***

In 2012, I had another mammogram. I was called back for a second mammogram which didn't bother me as much as it did before. I was getting used to this! After the second mammogram, I was sent home and was told that they would contact me if I needed any further testing.

About a week later, I received a piece of mail from the imaging center. When I opened it, my heart sank. They wanted me to return for further testing.

"Oh, no," I thought to myself. "What if they find cancer THIS time?"

I made the appointment and showed up for additional testing about a week later. The first thing they did was perform another mammogram. This time, the tech pressed those plates down so hard on my breast that I thought I was going to pass out. I had been through this before, and I knew it would only last a few seconds, so I closed my eyes and just prayed my way through it.

"OK, let me go show these to the radiologist. You can sit right here. I'll be back in a few minutes."

I looked around the dark room. "How many people have been in this very room as they received shocking news?" I thought to myself. "I hope I'm not going to be one of them."

I patiently waited and tried not to worry, but that is almost impossible. Every woman who goes through this knows that the chances are that everything is OK, but there is ALWAYS that chance that it will not be OK.

Finally, the tech returned.

"The radiologist wants an ultrasound," she said.

"Oh, OK," I said before I had time to think.

"Follow me," she said.

I followed her into another darkened room. There was a table with an ultrasound machine beside it.

"OK, lay down here on your back, and open your robe on your right side.

I felt a little uncomfortable as I lay there with my right breast exposed. She took a tube and squirted gel on my breast, picked up the probe attached to the machine, and started moving it around on my breast. I turned my head to the right and up to see the screen. I wanted to see what she was doing.

As she moved the probe, I saw little squiggly white lines with a dark gray background. It made absolutely no sense to someone who had no background in radiology. However, when she saw a large round like structure that looked completely dark gray, she stopped and took several pictures of it.

"Is that the thing that the radiologist is worried about?"

"Yep, that's it," she responded.

I didn't ask her what she thought it was because I knew that she would not be able to tell me even if she knew. I continued to watch, wondering if I was looking at cancer. She moved the probe around some more and took some additional pictures of smaller versions of that dark gray spot in my breast. I had multiple little spots like this throughout my breast.

"OK, I'm done," she said as she returned the probe to its holder. She handed me a towel.

"Wipe yourself off, and I'll be back."

I took the towel, cleaned myself up, and closed my robe. A few minutes later, the radiologist entered the room.

"Well, you have a lot of cysts in your breast," he said, "but no cancer. They are just cysts – some of them rather large."

I breathed deeply and said, "Thank God!"

"Now, I can drain those cysts if they are bothering you. That's up to you."

At that point in time, those cysts were not bothering me like they had in my 20s. Maybe it was because I was getting close to menopause. I thought a few seconds.

"No," I responded. "I think I'm OK for now."

"OK, no problem. If they start to bother you, we can drain them later."

"OK, good to know," I responded. "Thank you."

I left that day so incredibly happy that I didn't have cancer. I just had very lumpy breasts.

***

Around 2014, I officially entered menopause. The spotting that drove me crazy after my hysterectomy had ended, and I was so happy that I no longer had to wear panty liners. It was finally completely over!

Later that year, I pierced my ears for a 4th time. Finally, I was able to wear any earrings I wanted to wear! The rash did not reappear except on one day in 2021 when, for some reason, I broke out on my right earlobe. I didn't wear earrings for about a week, and the rash cleared up. Since then, I have worn earrings, and the rash has not returned. I assume this is because I am now through menopause, and my estrogen levels are low.

Around the same time, arthritis started to become a big problem for me. I had pain in multiple joints, and I felt tired all the time. I made an appointment with a rheumatologist who ran a battery of blood tests. I found out that my anti-nuclear antibody test (ANA) was low positive, and I tested low positive for scleroderma. I was shocked!

Although I tested positive for scleroderma, I did not have the clinical symptoms of the disorder, so I was never diagnosed with the condition. I was eventually diagnosed with fibromyalgia and undifferentiated connective tissue disease.

***

In the fall of 2017, I started to have episodes of nausea and gnawing pain especially after eating fatty meals. The episodes would last for several hours, but it wasn't horrible – just annoying. In November of that year, I had one particularly severe attack which landed me in the hospital.

My mom and I decided to go to a pancake breakfast that was being hosted by a local fire department. I had pancakes and a couple of sausage links. These sausage links were made by a local meat producer, and they were very tasty, so I went back for some more. A few hours later, I started to feel nauseated. I rested during the day, but the nausea didn't let up much. I ate very little the rest of the day.

The next morning, I woke up feeling terrible. I decided at that point that I needed to go to the hospital. My mom drove me there, and they performed blood tests and an ultrasound. The ultrasound showed a dilated pancreatic duct and gallstones. It was decided that I needed to have my gallbladder removed.

"Another surgery?" I thought to myself. I could not believe it. As I waited to be admitted, my mom and I counted how many surgeries that I had in my lifetime, and we counted 12. I just shook my head.

After the surgery, my surgeon told me that I had quite a few gallstones and that there was chronic scarring of the gallbladder. She was quite sure that this was what caused my nausea and gnawing pain in my abdomen.

She was right. After this surgery, those symptoms disappeared although I now must be careful about eating certain foods, especially greasy foods, as it can give me diarrhea. But that problem pales in comparison to the nausea I felt prior to surgery.

***

My right knee has been creaking and cracking since my 20s. It never really caused me significant problems, however, until 2018.

I had some imaging done on my knee in 2014 or so because it did hurt some, and the noise it was making sounded like my knee was crunching into a million pieces! The MRI showed that I had chondromalacia behind my kneecap along with a Baker's cyst. Even though these issues were found, I decided to forgo surgery at that time since the pain wasn't severe. Instead, I went to physical therapy which did help.

By 2018, the pain had gotten progressively worse, and my knee had been giving out on me. Another MRI was done, and in addition to what was found in 2014, a torn lateral meniscus was noted. I decided to go ahead with surgery which was done in 2019.

Prior to this surgery, the orthopedic surgeon and nurses had a long discussion about what antibiotic to give to me since I was allergic to so many. They finally decided on vancomycin. It was given to me slowly through a drip in my IV. My mom was with me during this surgery, and I joked around with her, telling her that if I turn bright red to make sure and get the nurse. I really didn't think anything was going to happen as the medical professionals discussed this at length before giving it to me, and they were giving it to me very slowly. About 20 minutes after starting the drip, my top of my head started to itch. At first, I didn't think much of it, but it quickly increased in intensity. I was clawing at my head, so my mom went to get the nurse. By the time they got back to me, I was bright red and was scratching my head like crazy. The nurse quickly turned off the drip. The orthopedic surgeon came in a few minutes later.

"Oh, wow," he said. "Red man syndrome."

I laughed as I thought he was making a joke. He didn't laugh. When I realized that he wasn't joking, I stopped laughing.

"What?" I asked.

"Red man syndrome," he repeated. "It's a well-known allergic reaction to vancomycin," he said as he checked my IV.

"Oh, you have got to be kidding me!" I exclaimed. "Another antibiotic allergy?"

"I'm afraid so," he said as he turned to the nurse. "Let's give her some IV Benadryl®."

Enough of the vancomycin had been given to me, so they didn't give me any other antibiotic at that time, but I was just in such disbelief that I was now not allowed to take five antibiotics due to allergic reactions!

***

At Christmas in 2019, after I did some low-impact exercises, I suddenly had severe right-sided pain. I felt something under my ribs on my right side make a snapping noise. I was convinced that I had broken a rib, so I went to the emergency room. An x-ray did not pick up any break, so I was told that I probably pulled or tore a muscle or tendon. I was sent home with pain medication and was told to rest at home to allow it to heal.

Two days later, I went to bed after watching all my favorite TV shows. It was just like any other night. I got in bed, and I sat up to adjust my sheet when suddenly, a huge wave of pain traveled across my abdomen under my right ribs. I slowly laid down and quickly realized that I was much more comfortable laying on my left side. I thought at the time that I pulled the muscle or tendon again, so I just laid there, hoping the pain would subside. At one point during the night, I tried to roll over on my right side, but the pain was so intense that I could not stand it. Finally, at around 6 a.m., I called the ambulance.

I patiently waited in the ER for the doctor to see me. I felt horrible. Finally, the doctor came into my room and examined me. She told the nurse to give me pain medication, and she ordered a lot of bloodwork. It was difficult for me to move, but I had to in order to get my blood drawn. The pain was unrelenting. Not even 30 minutes later, the doctor came rushing into the room.

"We are admitting you," she said.

Shocked, I responded, "What? What's wrong?"

"Your bloodwork shows that you have extremely elevated liver enzymes and abnormal pancreatic tests."

"What does that mean?" I asked as several nurses unlocked my bed in preparation to move it.

"We don't know yet," she responded. "Do you drink a lot of alcohol?"

"Oh, no," I responded. "I think I've had maybe two glasses of wine all year."

"OK," she responded. "It might be a gallstone. We'll have to do more tests to see where the problem is."

The nurse started to move my bed out of the room. I was in complete shock.

I ended up being hospitalized for a week. I had an endoscopy which didn't show much other than a very dilated pancreatic duct. When my lipase level increased to over 3,000 U/L (normal level is 0 – 160 U/L), I was transferred to another hospital where they had the capability to perform a test called an endoscopic retrograde cholangiopancreatography (ERCP). By the time this test was done, the swelling and/inflammation had gone down.

The doctor who performed the test thought that it was a gallstone; however, the gallstone was never seen, so this was just a guess. They think the gallstone passed through my system before these tests were performed. Since this happened, I have had no liver/pancreas issues again, so I hope this was just a one-time event.

I do want to share one specific story that occurred during my hospitalization for pancreatitis. One day, a nurse came in and talked to me as she changed my IV bag. She saw that my diagnosis was pancreatitis.

"Oh, pancreatitis!" she said. "You know that is supposed to be one of the most painful conditions!"

"Really?" I asked.

"Oh yes. It's supposed to be awful."

I never forgot that. Pancreatitis is one of the most painful conditions? Really? I can tell you with certainty that adenomyosis and endometriosis are FAR more painful than pancreatitis. Also, adenomyosis and endometriosis are more painful than a ruptured appendix.

On a scale of 1 to 10 (1 being little pain and 10 being the most painful), this is how I would rate the three above conditions in my case:

- Adenomyosis/endometriosis – 10
- Appendicitis – 8
- Pancreatitis – 6

I strongly believe that most doctors/friends/family members have no idea – not an inkling – of the degree of pain that adenomyosis and endometriosis patients must tolerate. In my book, *The Women Speak*, many women say the pain of adenomyosis is comparable to labor pain. I have never given birth, so I do not have a frame of reference personally, but some of the women in my support group who have gone through NATURAL childbirth say their pain from adenomyosis is WORSE than that. This disorder is extremely painful – far worse than normal period cramps.

***

Since I am so allergic to antibiotics, my allergist agreed to perform a test to see if I was truly allergic to penicillin. The nurse explained to me that many people in my age group who were told they were allergic to penicillin were not actually allergic to it. The rash may have been due to the virus we were fighting and not due an actual drug reaction.

During the test, I was given increasing amounts of amoxicillin over a 3-hour period, and thankfully, I did not react. He explained that I could take penicillin/amoxicillin and I would not have a type I allergic reaction (anaphylaxis). I may get a rash, but it would not progress to anaphylaxis. I am so glad that I have this information as it gives another possible antibiotic that I can take just in case I need it.

I may need another knee surgery as I have two more tears in the meniscus in my right knee. Since there are so many issues with this knee, the possibility of knee replacement has been discussed. However, we are not at that point yet.

While researching for this book, I found several clinical studies that found that women with endometriosis and adenomyosis may have low cortisol levels. Intrigued by this, I ordered a salivary cortisol test through Everlywell®. I was doubtful that it would come back abnormal since I had already entered menopause; however, I do have trouble with extreme fatigue today which is a symptom of low cortisol (but it could be a symptom of many other things as well). Anyway, not really expecting much from this test, I sent it in, and I am so glad I did. My salivary cortisol was extremely low at 0.6 ng/ml (normal values are 1.5-9.6 ng/ml).

Ninety percent of cortisol is bound to corticosteroid-binding globulin (CBG), also known as transcortin. Only about 10 percent is free cortisol, and it is this free cortisol that enters cells where is exerts its influence. Serum cortisol testing (through a blood sample) tests total cortisol levels (both free cortisol and cortisol bound to CBG) while salivary cortisol only tests levels of free cortisol. Therefore, many scientists opine that salivary testing of cortisol levels gives a more accurate picture of the actual activity of cortisol in the body.

My family doctor referred me to an endocrinologist for further testing. This endocrinologist order both serum cortisol testing (total cortisol) and salivary cortisol testing (free cortisol). The salivary cortisol involved 2 samples – one taken upon awakening, and the other taken 60 minutes later. She also tested ACTH levels. All tests were performed by Quest Diagnostics®.

Serum cortisol (total cortisol) and ACTH levels were normal. However, my salivary cortisol (free cortisol) upon awakening was twice as high as it should have been at 1.09 mcg/dl (normal range is 0.04-0.56 mcg/dl). Sixty minutes later, the value dropped to within normal range at 0.41 mcg/dl. This initial increase and drop in cortisol, known as the cortisol awakening response, is normal. However, I still wonder why my awakening level was so high.

It is important to note that the saliva tests were done by two different labs. The saliva test done through Everlywell® was not an awakening cortisol level. I had been awake for about an hour before I performed the test. Everlywell® required saliva that I spit into a tube, while Quest Diagnostics® used a Salivette® tube in which I had to roll a large cotton-type swab around in my mouth for several minutes. Differences in the times the tests were performed could partially explain the differences in the results.

Although I do not fully understand why the results are so different, I think it is important to note that the salivary cortisol results from both labs were significantly out of range – one was too low, and the other was too high. Could there be more to this story? Possibly.

Multiple studies have examined cortisol levels in both salivary and serum samples in women with endometriosis. In 2002, Smith et al. reported that total cortisol concentration in follicular fluid in women with minimal to mild endometriosis were significantly lower than in controls. However, Lima et al. (2006) looked at cortisol and prolactin levels in serum, peritoneal, and follicular fluid from infertile women with endometriosis and those levels to levels in women who were fertile and who did not have endometriosis. They found that the levels of cortisol in peritoneal and follicular fluid was not significantly different between the two groups, but the serum cortisol levels were significantly higher in the endometriosis group. They state, "Since higher levels of cortisol and prolactin are often associated with stress, it is probable that stress might contribute to the development of endometriosis and its progression to advanced stages of the disease."

In 2008, Petrelluzzi et al. found low salivary cortisol levels in endometriosis patients. They concluded, "Women with endometriosis and chronic pelvic pain show low concentrations of salivary cortisol and a high level of perceived stress associated with a poor quality of life." Quinones et al. (2015) looked at 32 salivary samples from patients with endometriosis and compared these levels to 36 healthy controls. The researchers found that incapacitating pain was a strong predictor of low cortisol levels. They state, "This study supports previous reports of hypocortisolism as a biomarker of aberrant [hypothalamus-pituitary-adrenal] responses in women with endometriosis." In 2021, Vanuccini et al. discussed abnormalities in the hypothalamus-pituitary-adrenal axis in women with endometriosis. They state, "A paradoxical hypocortisolism like an adrenal fatigue may exacerbate painful symptoms by reducing the endogenous analgesia associated with stress…"

Although, hypocortisolism has been reported multiple times in women with endometriosis, more studies need to be done. Considering the results of studies and the odd cortisol levels in my own testing, I think it is very important to evaluate these levels in patients with adenomyosis and/or endometriosis. I believe the adrenal glands have been largely ignored by gynecologists when evaluating these patients. We must remember that the adrenal glands are intricately intertwined with the hypothalamus and pituitary gland, and all three glands are involved in the regulation of reproductive hormones.

Today, I still struggle with pain from arthritis – arthritis in my lower back, arthritis in my knee, arthritis in my hip, and even the occasional flare-up of pain in my neck which is due to several bulging discs that probably developed because of looking through a microscope for so many years. I have been diagnosed with fibromyalgia and undifferentiated connective tissue disease. I am currently on gabapentin for pain from arthritis, and I take the antidepressant Effexor® (venlafaxine) for depression. In addition, I take Singulair® and Flonase® in order to keep my allergies at bay in addition to receiving monthly allergy shots. I now take prescription vitamin D continually since I am not able to keep my level in the normal range.

I am also in physical therapy multiple times a year. This helps in keeping my arthritis pain under control. I do not want to have any more spinal surgeries if possible. Additionally, I have to be very careful to not eat fatty foods as those types of foods can cause nausea, diarrhea, and acid reflux because my gallbladder is gone. However, the good news is that the pain and heavy bleeding that I suffered from for seventeen years is finally gone...for good!

Part II – Adenomyosis and Endometriosis – What We Know Today

Basics of Endometriosis

"Endometriosis is "an inflammatory disease process characterized at surgery by the presence of endometrium-like epithelium and/or stroma outside the endometrium and myometrium..."

-Center for Endometriosis Care

Endometriosis occurs when endometrial-like implants are present outside the uterus, commonly on the ovaries, bowel, and bladder. It is an estrogen-dependent disease. Endometriosis can cause severe abdominal pain, infertility, painful intercourse, back pain, leg and hip pain, painful bowel movements, and bladder dysfunction. These implants respond to hormonal stimulation and bleed during menstruation. Since the trapped blood has nowhere to go, this can cause inflammation which irritate nerves and cause severe pain in this disorder.

According to Dr. Camran Nezhat (2021), endometriosis is estimated to affect 200 million women and girls around the world, and it takes on average 6 to 10 years to get accurately diagnosed. He also states that a study cited endometriosis as being one of the top ten most painful conditions. In addition, this disorder is commonly undiagnosed because of medical myths such as the belief that the pain is normal.

The American Society of Reproductive Medicine has established a classification system for endometriosis. However, it is important to remember that the degree of the disease does not correlate with the degree of pain felt by the patient. For example, a patient with stage 4 disease may not have much pain while a patient with stage 1 disease may have excruciating pain. The following is the classification system:

- Stage 1- minimal disease
- Stage 2 – mild disease
- Stage 3 – moderate disease

- Stage 4 – severe disease

According to the Center for Innovative GYN Care (CIGC, 2021), pain in the back, legs, and hips can occur if lesions affect the sciatic nerve. They also state that lesions on the bowel can cause severe pain, painful bowel movements, constipation, and/or diarrhea which many times leads to the misdiagnosis of IBS. In addition, these physicians talk about pain during sex. They state, "In some cases, certain positions can cause sharp or stabbing pain if endometriosis lesions are present around the uterus, cervix, or bowel."

Other symptoms of endometriosis include bloating, nausea, and painful ovulation. Sometimes, abdominal bloating may lead to the impression that the patient has gained weight or is pregnant. Nausea and vomiting can occur because of the severe pain associated with endometriosis. Painful ovulation can occur when lesions are present on the ovaries.

Endometriosis can also form adhesions in the pelvic region. Adhesions are bands of scar tissue that bind two organs together and can cause severe pain. See Adhesions section for more information.

The following are the symptoms of endometriosis:

- Dysmenorrhea (painful menstrual cramps)
- Dyspareunia (painful intercourse) - can occur during or after sex
- Inability to insert tampons due to pain
- Heavy menstrual bleeding
- Painful urination during menstruation
- Painful bowel movements during menstruation
- Infertility
- Nausea
- Diarrhea and/or constipation
- Spotting/bleeding between periods

- Fatigue
- Bloating
- Allergies
- Migraines
- Leg and/or lower back pain

According to the Center for Endometriosis Care, there are currently no available blood tests or biomarkers for endometriosis. Many are being tested, but none have proved efficacious at this time.

Basics of Adenomyosis

"Courage does not always roar. Sometimes courage is the quiet voice at the end of the day saying, 'I will try again tomorrow.'"

-Mary Anne Radmacher

Dr. Eisen Liang from the Sydney Fibroid Clinic in Sydney Australia accurately describes adenomyosis as "the (bad) cousin of endometriosis." These two conditions are similar but also have some very distinct differences.

Adenomyosis has been referred to as "endometriosis interna." The reason for this is because endometrial-like tissue is located within the muscle of the uterine wall (myometrium) in adenomyosis whereas this kind of tissue occurs outside of the uterus in endometriosis. To complicate matters, the symptoms of adenomyosis and endometriosis are similar, and the ability to distinguish between the two requires expertise on the part of physicians and sonographers/radiologists who are well-trained in the two disorders.

As Dr. Liang (2021) states in his book, *Could it be Adenomyosis? The (Bad) Cousin of Endometriosis*, one significant difference between the two conditions is that endometriosis patients typically suffer from dysmenorrhea (period pain). Adenomyosis typically presents with dysmenorrhea and menorrhagia (heavy menstrual bleeding). However, endometriosis patients can also suffer from menorrhagia.

Adenomyosis can be difficult to pick up if the sonographer/radiologist is not properly trained. Some of the features of adenomyosis are subtle on ultrasound. The condition is more easily seen on MRI.

In many cases, adenomyosis and endometriosis occur together. Kunz et al. (2007) state adenomyosis and endometriosis may be different forms of the same disease since both involve displaced endometrial-like tissue. In addition, these same investigators determined that in a group of women with known endometriosis, 70% also had adenomyosis as compared to a control group in which only 9% of women were found to have the disorder. Although convincing, another group of researchers, Bazot et al. (2001) only found 27% of women with endometriosis had adenomyosis. The discrepancy can be blamed on the different imaging criteria used to diagnose the disorders. Dr. Albee at the Center for Endometriosis Care (2017) states, "In my experience at the Center for Endometriosis Care, every time a patient has requested hysterectomy after conservative surgery for endometriosis failed to control severe dysmenorrhea (cramps) or central pelvic pain, adenomyosis has been found in the uterus."

The symptoms of adenomyosis are as follows:

- Painful menstrual bleeding (dysmenorrhea) – cramping may be as severe as the last stage of labor
- Heavy menstrual bleeding (menorrhagia)
- Prolonged menstrual bleeding (more than 10 days) or non-stop bleeding
- Enlarged, heavy, and bulky uterus (often doubling or tripling in size) that leads to severe bloating
- Tenderness or pain during a pelvic exam
- A "bearing down" sensation
- Heaviness and/or pain in the legs
- Spotting or bleeding between periods
- Painful intercourse (dyspareunia)
- Pressure on the bladder
- Painful bowel movements during menstruation
- Passing large and/or many blood clots – size can be anywhere from the size of a dime to as large as the palm of hand
- Chronic anemia due to excessive blood loss resulting in debilitating fatigue

- Depression and/or anxiety
- Infertility
- Increase in debilitating pain over time
- More common as women get older

**Some women have no symptoms

Adhesions

"Best medicine in the world? Listening to the patient."

-Dr. Camran Nezhat

Adhesions are scar tissue that binds two organs together and leads to pain and other issues. When endometriosis lesions bleed in the pelvis during menstruation, this leads to inflammation which can lead to the development of adhesions. The same type of phenomenon can occur during surgery according to Dr. Ken Sinervo (2021). Any intra-abdominal blood can lead to the formation of adhesions. Therefore, surgical technique during endometriosis excision and other abdominal surgeries is vitally important to prevent adhesion formation.

Adhesions can cause painful bowel symptoms such as constipation, diarrhea, and difficult/painful bowel movements (dyschezia). According to Dr. Ken Sinervo (2021), adhesions can bind the bowel to ovaries, uterus and even the pelvic sidewall. In addition, adhesions can be one of the causes of abdominal bloating. According to Dr. Tamer Seckin (2020), "This is fibrosis. It's important to understand what adhesions are because adhesions in a large scale can cause intestinal obstruction."

Adhesions can be removed, but this kind of surgery should only be performed by laparoscopic surgeons that are specifically experienced and trained in this type of surgery.

Symptoms of adhesions can include the following:

- Dyspareunia (painful intercourse)
- Infertility
- Constipation
- Diarrhea

- Intestinal obstruction
- Pelvic pain
- Dyschezia

Allergies

"Although there is information on the relationship of hormones, allergy, and autoimmune diseases, this relationship is, however, poorly understood."

-Shilpa Shah

Women with endometriosis tend to have an increased risk of developing autoimmune diseases and allergies, especially asthma. According to Caserta et al. (2015), "The possible involvement of the immune system in the pathogenesis of endometriosis and coexistence of diseases that involve the immune system such as allergies, asthma, and autoimmune diseases, seem to be related."

Most of our immune cells express estrogen receptors, specifically estrogen receptor alpha (ERα) and estrogen receptor beta (ERβ). These immune cells can respond to estrogen to varying degrees. Therefore, estrogen can exert effects on our immune system which could lead to allergic reactions.

Allergic reactions, specifically asthma, have been shown to be exacerbated during PMS. Keselman and Heller (2015) state, "Roughly 33-52% of asthmatic women report premenstrual worsening of symptoms" and "Almost 50% of women hospitalized for asthma symptoms are identified as premenstrual." In addition, these researchers point out, "The incidence of allergy and asthma peaks in women after puberty and strongly subsides with age."

To understand the rest of this section, it is important to understand the basics of how our immune system works. This is a very complicated topic, so this will be just a basic explanation. First, let's start with some definitions.

There are multiple types of immunity, but we are going to start with the basics. Innate immunity is present at birth. This type of immunity lasts a lifetime and are typically the first responders when a pathogen invades the body. Adaptive immunity are specialized immune cells that attack foreign invaders and then remember these invaders in case a future infection occurs. An antigen is a foreign substance such as a bacteria or a virus. A "foreign invader" is also referred to as an antigen.

Lymphocytes are very important cells found in the lymph and blood. The two main types are B-cells and T-cells.

T-cells are part of our immune system and are part of our adaptive immunity. They are produced in the thymus gland. Once released from the thymus, they circulate throughout the body until they encounter an antigen-presenting cell (APC) described below. When T-cells mature, they develop into T-helper cells, T-cytotoxic cells, memory T-cells, and regulatory T-cells. T-cells are involved in cell-mediated immunity. This is a type of immune response that does not involve antibodies (see B-cells below). Instead this type of response involves the activation of cytotoxic T-cells and phagocytosis (explained below).

B-cells produce antibodies, also known as immunoglobulins, after they come in contact with an antigen. When this occurs, the B-cell divided and clones itself which results in millions of these antibodies being released into the bloodstream and lymph tissue. B-cells recognize free antigen, but they will not activate until it receives a signal from T-helper cells.

Macrophages are large white blood cells that engulf antigens. In my microbiology classes in college, I always imagined them as "Pac Man". They go throughout the body just eating up things that aren't supposed to be there. This process is called phagocytosis. These cells are a part of our innate immune system.

Natural killer (NK) cells are part of our innate immunity, and they are usually the first responders of our immune system. Dendritic cells activate T and B lymphocytes.

Eosinophils are a type of white blood cell that are active in allergy and asthma. They release inflammatory molecules and cytotoxic proteins. Mast cells release histamine to help get rid of allergens.

Now that we have the basic definitions, let's take a basic look at how all of these different cells interact.

First, an antigen (a foreign substance) encounters our immune cells such as macrophages and T helper cells. T helper cells are further subdivided into Th1 and Th2 cells. Th1 responses are generally directed at viruses and bacteria. Th2 responses are typically directed at allergens and helminths (parasitic worms). When antigens encounter our immune cells, it binds to them, and the immune cells become activated. These activated cells are called antigen-presenting cells, or APCs. Helper T-cells also secrete cytokines, as described below, that help B-cells differentiate into plasma cells. They are also involved in the activation of cytotoxic T-cells and macrophages.

There are 3 types of APCs – dendritic cells, activated macrophages, and B-lymphocytes. As stated before, B-cells recognize antigen but are not activated until they receive a signal from the T-cells, specifically, Th2. Cytokines released from Th2 cells diffuse into the B cells which then lead to the production of antibodies.

Cytokines are small proteins involved in cell signaling and are vital in the proper functioning of the immune system. The interleukins, interferon, TNF, and chemokines are all types of cytokines. The cytokines produced during a Th2 response include interleukin 4 (IL-4), interleukin 5 (IL-5), and interleukin 13 (IL-13), and these are associated with the production of immunoglobulin E (IgE) which leads to allergic symptoms.

Interleukin 12 (IL-12) is produced by activated macrophages. This interleukin induces Th1 differentiation which leads to cell-mediated immunity. In addition to IL-12, other factors are involved in cell-mediated immunity such as tumor necrosis factor alpha (TNF-α), interferon gamma (IFN-gamma which is derived from natural killer cells, aka NK cells) These stimulate the activity of T cytotoxic cells, NK cells, and activated macrophages.

One of the first studies that linked hormone levels and allergies was conducted by Roby et al. in 2006. They examined progesterone and estrogen antibody levels in patients that had menstrual-related complaints such as migraine, asthma, and joint pain. These patients had higher estrogen and progesterone antibodies (IgG, IgM, and IgE) than those women without menstrual related complaints.

Shilpa Shah (2012) studied the possibility of a hormonal link to autoimmune allergies. He points out that there is a "disproportionate representation of males before puberty and females after puberty" when it comes to allergy and autoimmune diseases. This indicates that there is a role for sex hormones in these diseases.

Shah (2012) explains how a hormone allergy can occur. Estrogen, progesterone, and their metabolites may act as antigens. This promotes the development of Th2 cells which regulates the synthesis of antibodies and IgE. These antibodies then bind to mast cells which induce mast cell degranulation. This leads to histamine release resulting in a Type I allergic reaction. Another possibility is a Type IV allergic reaction that is predominately regulated through Th1. This can occur when the hormones bind to blood proteins. Lymphocytes will react to this complex, inducing cytokine production and lymphocyte proliferation.

As stated above, IgE production leads to allergic symptoms via the Th2 response. This happens when an allergic individual is exposed to an exogenous allergen (for example, pollen). However, Shah (2012) suggests that when a person has allergic symptoms without exposure to the exogenous allergen, this might resemble a Th1 chronic inflammatory reaction which may lead to autoimmune allergies.

Caserta et al. (2015) points out that Th2 responses counteract Th1 responses. Because of this, they conclude that "...the high incidence of allergies in the endometriosis group could be explained by the inhibitory effect on Th1. The inhibition of Th1 would reduce NK cells, which would lead to an impaired clearing of endometrial cells, playing a fundamental role in endometriosis." The researchers go on to say, "...many studies have been performed which stress different alterations of the immune components of the suffering women, such as a function anomaly of the T and B lymphocytes and the attendant high serum levels of IgG, IgA, and IgM, but contemporary reduction of the activity of the natural killer (NK) cells."

Kalogeromitros et al. (1995) reported skin prick testing on women during days 12 to 16 of their cycles showed significantly increased wheel-and-flare responses. Interestingly, estrogen levels are at their peak during this time. Kirmaz et al. (2004) confirmed the estrogen link with allergies and found that luteinizing hormone (LH) levels were high and correlated with increased skin-prick reactions at midcycle. In addition, Haeggstrom et al. (2000) showed that the peak levels of estrogen during the menstrual cycle affected the nasal mucosa by making it hyperactive to histamine.

Sinaii et al. (2002) showed that allergies, fibromyalgia, chronic fatigue syndrome, hypothyroidism and other autoimmune disorders are higher among women with endometriosis when compared to the general population. The following chart shows the actual numbers:

Endometriosis   General Population

Hypothyroidism	9.6%	1.5%
Fibromyalgia	5.9%	3.4%
Chronic fatigue	4.6%	.03%
Rheumatoid arthritis	1.8%	1.2%
Sjogren's syndrome	.6%	.03%
Multiple sclerosis	.5%	.07%

No connection was found between endometriosis and hyperthyroidism or diabetes.

Sinaii et all. (2002) also explains why endometriosis may have an autoimmune factor at play as it has been shown that this disease has high T- and B-lymphocyte counts, high serum levels of IgG, IgM and IgA autoantibodies, anti-endometrial antibodies, and a reduced natural killer cell activity. In addition, they state that allergies, eczema, and asthma may be more common in endometriosis due to the presence of degranulating eosinophils and eotaxin (a type of chemokine that attracts eosinophils).

Matalliotakis et al. (2012) evaluated 501 women with endometriosis and 188 women without the disease at Yale University Hospital. They were able to show a link between endometriosis and an increased risk of allergic autoimmune disorders. They state, "...women with endometriosis were significantly more likely to report a positive family history of allergies."

According to Shah (2012), the following are symptoms of a hormone allergy. In my case, I had 11 out of 15 of these symptoms:

- Premenstrual syndrome
- Premenstrual asthma
- Menstrual migraines
- Weight problems

- Loss of short-term memory
- Fatigue
- Skin problems
- Mood swings
- Diminished sex drive
- Anxiety and panic attacks
- Fibromyalgia
- Interstitial cystitis
- Arthritis
- Chronic fatigue syndrome
- Infertility

In addition to the above list, Untersmayr et al. (2017) stated that dermatitis, dysmenorrhea, rhinitis, itching, and bullous erythema may also be indicators of hormone allergy. Specifically, they state, "...dermal manifestations range from itching, urticaria, eczema, papillo-vesicular or vesiculobullous dermatosis, erythema multiforme, hirsutism with or without acne and hyperpigmentation, purpura, and petechiae to stomatitis."

In addition to the above allergies, nickel allergy has been shown to be a possible risk factor for endometriosis. A study done by Yuk et al. (2015) in South Korea showed this link in their study. They evaluated 4,985 women of which 997 women had endometriosis and 3988 women without endometriosis served as the control group. 0.8% of the women with endometriosis had a nickel allergy while only 0.3% of the women in the control group were allergic to nickel. Silva et al. (2013) showed that nickel concentrations in the blood of women with endometriosis were higher than in women without the disease. Interestingly, according to Yuk et al. (2015), "the occurrence of nickel allergy increases with exposure to nickel."

Borghini et al (2020) showed that 90% of endometriosis patients were positive for nickel sensitivity. It has also been shown that nickel sensitivity in endometriosis patients is correlated with

IBS-like symptoms. They found that after three months on a low nickel diet, the test group showed a statistically significant reduction of gastrointestinal, extra-intestinal and gynecological symptoms. The group concluded that a low nickel diet "may be recommended in this condition to reduce gastrointestinal, extra-intestinal and gynecological symptoms."

There is some evidence that nickel has estrogenic properties. Medici et al. (1989) showed that nickel can bind to sites on the estrogen receptor in the calf uterus. Martin et al. (2003) was able to show that nickel can stimulate ERα expression and activity in breast cancer cells. Therefore, this estrogenic activity of nickel could play a role in the development of endometriosis and adenomyosis. More studies are needed to determine the role of nickel in the development of these disorders.

This past year, as I wrote this book, I decided to set up a poll on the Adenomyosis Fighters Support Group Facebook page and asked members what allergies they had. There were 1,210 responses. I was intrigued by the responses. Eleven members reported having mast cell disorders including mast cell activation syndrome. In addition, 36 members report having histamine intolerance. These findings suggest a possible role of the immune system in these disorders. Additional clinical studies would be very helpful to see if the immune system is involved and exactly how the immune system is linked to these disorders.

In those with food allergies, there appears to be a fair number with allergies to fruit. I wonder if the allergy is to the fruit or to whatever pesticide is being sprayed on the fruit. Again, additional clinical studies are desperately needed. I also found it fascinating that almost 100 respondents had antibiotic allergies just like me, and what I found even more interesting was that 10 respondents report an allergy to sulfa. Surprisingly, only 19 members report having a nickel allergy. The results are below:

Any kind of tree	178
Grasses or weeds	145

Dust	140	
Mold	106	
Food allergies	102	
(10 allergic to kiwi, 10 allergic to pineapple, 4 allergic to stone fruit)		
Animals		101
Antibiotics	97	
(10 allergic to sulfa antibiotics)		
Autoimmune disease	70	
Insect stings	40	
Histamine intolerance	36	
Dust mites	33	
Latex	27	
Poison ivy/poison oak	20	
Nickel	19	
Adhesives	13	
NSAIDS		13
Mast cell disorder (MCAS)	11	
Vicodin	5	
Gluten	4	
Other	4	
Acetaminophen	2	

** 17 members report no known allergies

Interestingly, in my case, my family has an extraordinarily strong history of allergy, especially in my maternal grandmother. I never knew her as she passed away from breast cancer before I was born (she was only 41 years old), but my uncles told me that she had terrible asthma and allergies. In fact, every spring, they would take her from Kentucky to Michigan during the height of the allergy season to give her a reprieve from her symptoms. Additionally, my mom and siblings also have a history of significant allergies; however, none of us have asthma. The above studies show a strong correlation between hormone levels and allergies, and this explains a lot in my case of PMS allergies and nickel allergy.

Aromatase Inhibitors

"You can think of your body's many hormones as part of an elaborate messenger system, dashing through your bloodstream to share information, give instructions, and coordinate functions among your organs and nervous system."

-Marcelle Pick from her book, *Is it Me or My Hormones?*

In both endometriosis and adenomyosis, there is increased activity of the enzyme aromatase. This enzyme increases the ability of androgens, such as testosterone, to convert to estrogen.

Endometriosis and adenomyosis are known to be estrogen-dependent disorders, and the locally produced estrogen in these disorders has been shown to be the more potent estrogen called estradiol (E2). This elevated production of E2 has been attributed to a defect in the function of stromal cells involving the enzyme 17β-HSD-2. This enzyme catalyzes the conversion of the more potent E2 to the weaker estrogen E1 (estrone). In addition, according to Pamela Smith (2010), the expression of 17β-hydroxysteroid type 2 (17-β-HSD type 2) is deficient in endometriosis.

It has been found that in endometriosis and adenomyosis, there is progesterone resistance. Progesterone stimulates the production of 17β-HSD type 2. Because there is progesterone resistance and low progesterone production in these disorders, 17β-HSD type 2 is deficient which leaves excess E2 present in a woman's body. In addition, estrogen upregulates the production of prostaglandin E2 (PGE2). PGE2 is a known potent inducer of aromatase activity.

The following are factors known to increase aromatase levels:

- Elevated insulin
- Elevated cortisol

- Being overweight
- Inflammation

Flaxseed, grape seed extract, and red wine have all been shown to reduce aromatase levels which may partly explain why my symptoms improved once I added flaxseed to my diet.

In a study done by Soysal et al. (2004), the use of aromatase inhibitors in addition to GnRH agonists in women with endometriosis showed promising results as it reduced the risk of recurrence for 24 months. Kimura et al. (2007) confirmed this finding and stated that this course of treatment may be useful in cases that were resistant to conventional treatments or in women who didn't want to have surgery. In addition, Badawy et al. (2012) showed that aromatase inhibitors are effective in reducing the size of adenomyomas and improving symptoms in affected women.

Aromatase inhibitors may be an effective treatment option for women with adenomyosis and endometriosis.

Bloating

"Symptoms are then in reality nothing but the cry from suffering organs."

-Jean Martin Charcot

The bloating associated with endometriosis is often referred to as "endo belly." This type of bloating is not the typical PMS bloating that some women experience. "Endo belly" refers to excessive bloating that makes a women look up to 9 months pregnant in some cases. It is also associated with severe pain that can be as severe as labor.

Dr. Sophie Chung, in an article written by Megan Seligman in 2021 for the Endometriosis Foundation of America, states that bloating may be caused by inflammation due to endometrial implants in the pelvis, small intestinal bacterial overgrowth (SIBO), fibroids, constipation, and/or gas.

"Endo belly" is quite common in women with endometriosis. Although in my case, the bloating occurred mostly at the end of my period, this bloating can occur at any time (not just menstruation). Griffiths, Koutsouridou and Penketh (2007) found that abdominal bloating was a strong marker for rectovaginal endometriosis which is what I suspect I had.

Moradi et al. (2019) found that 91.25% of endometriosis patients reported bloating as a symptom. Maroun et al. (2009) found that 90% of endometriosis patients in their study reported gastrointestinal symptoms. 82.8% of them specifically reported bloating. Sinaii et al. (2002) reported that 84% of the endometriosis patients in their study had bloating compared to the 12-16% of the general population that report bloating. Recently, I published a book that had results of questionnaires that I had posted on the Adenomyosis Fighters Support Group Facebook page. The percentage of women reported bloating as bad to extreme was 71.3 %. "Bad" indicated bloating to the size of a 4 to 5-month pregnancy. "Extreme" indicated bloating to the size of a 6 or more-month pregnancy. Interestingly, this group of women also reported problems eating during the time that they were bloated, and they also reported that the bloating worsened as the day progressed.

Bloating is a significant issue in both adenomyosis and endometriosis and has a detrimental effect on the quality of life in these women.

Colorectal Resection

"You are you because you love the way the world looks through your camera. You are you because of the way you love your friends and family. Not because some scar is on your body. That's a part of your history and what helps for what you believe in, not what defines you.

-A.M. Willard

In cases of deep infiltrating endometriosis (DIE), a bowel resection may be necessary. Deep infiltrating endometriosis refers to advanced endometriosis that has deeply invaded organs in the pelvic cavity and causes rectovaginal nodules in the cul-de-sac region.

Two surgical procedures are used. The first one involves removing an entire section of the colon and the rectum. The other approach only removes a section of the colon but does not involve the rectum.

The two major complications that may occur during a bowel resection are leakage occurring where the two sections of the bowel are reattached (anastomotic leakage) and rectovaginal fistula. Other complications include damage to the ureters, pelvic abscess, stricture of the colon at the surgical site, and postoperative bleeding.

A study by Ruffo et al (2014) regarding the long-term outcomes of bowel resections in cases of DIE concluded "The present results confirm that bowel resections for endometriosis are correlated with an acceptable complication rate even at long-term follow-up and that symptoms significantly improve over time, except for rectal bleeding and dysuria, the latter associated with a neurological damage." This study evaluated 900 patients with a median follow-up time of 54 months.

However, a French study by Roman et al. (2018) reviewed 60 cases of colorectal resection for treatment of DIE and found that these two types of resections end up with the same rate of bowel disorders after surgery. Thirteen women in each group reported some kind of bowel problem two years after surgery in this study.

If a woman has DIE and is faced with a colorectal resection, it is vitally important to get treatment from a surgeon who is well-trained in this kind of surgical procedure and who is well-versed in endometriosis. Refer to Recommended Treatment Facilities for names of top surgeons who have extensive experience in this kind of surgery.

Dyspareunia

"It is not OK to miss a part of your life because of pain and excessive bleeding. It is not OK to be bed-ridden for two to three days a month. It is not OK to have pain during sex. It is not OK to have major bloating or nausea."

-Susan Sarandon

Dyspareunia refers to painful sexual intercourse. According to Vercillini et al. (2012), women with endometriosis have a ninefold increase of experiencing painful sexual intercourse as compared to women in the general population of the same age.

Caserta et al. (2015) describe the symptoms as follows:

> "...pain with penetration more or less deep, with sexual intercourse, associated with pressure on the endometriotic nodules and on deep lesions infiltrating the uterus-sacral and cardinal ligaments, the [pouch of] Douglas, the posterior fornix of the vagina, and the anterior rectal wall..."

Moradi et al. (2014) performed a focal group study in which the participants talked about their experiences of living with endometriosis. Dyspareunia was a symptom in most of the participants, and they said the pain occurred during or after sex. One participant stated, "I started to worry when my ex-partner and I got together and the pain during and after sex just got that bad that I would just lay in a fetal position for hours afterwards...I would actually be crying during and after sex." Another participant stated, "The psychological damage that [this] has caused me is immense...I feel like I'm not even a woman...I feel like I'm denied some part of being human." The researchers stated that issues involved the following:

- Decrease in frequency of intercourse

- Avoiding sex due to pain or bleeding
- Failure to achieve orgasm

In addition, these researchers stated that these sexual problems led to relationship breakdowns for some of these women.

Vercillini et al. (2012) state that the pain may be caused traction of scarred tissue, immobilization of uterine pelvic structures, and pressure on the endometriotic nodules. This group performed a case control study comparing women with rectovaginal endometriosis, peritoneal and/or ovarian endometriosis and women without endometriosis (control group). They found that the women in the rectovaginal endometriosis (RVE) group suffered more from painful intercourse than women in either of the two other groups. They also noted that women with either RVE or peritoneal and/or ovarian endometriosis had poorer sexual functioning than women without endometriosis. These researchers also noted that "...sexual functioning in the immediate years after coitarche was very similar among the three study groups, suggesting that sexual dysfunction in women with rectovaginal endometriosis arose and increased during time, most probably as a result of the development of deep lesions."

For more information, see "Rectovaginal endometriosis."

Endometrial ablation

"Do not spend your precious energy worrying about how others view your medical condition.

-Toni Bernhard

Performed under general anesthesia, an endometrial ablation destroys the endometrial layer of the uterus.

The procedure can be done many ways using extreme cold, heated liquids, microwave energy, radiofrequency or electrosurgery. An endometrial ablation is not recommended for patients in the following circumstances:

- Those who wish to become pregnant in the future
- Those who have known uterine cancer
- Those who have recently had a baby
- Those who are post-menopausal

For those women who still wish to have children, endometrial ablation is not a practical option because this procedure damages the lining of the uterus. Although periods usually stop after this surgery, there have still been reports of pregnancy occurring after an endometrial ablation. These pregnancies usually end in miscarriage.

An incision is not necessary during this procedure. The tools required for an endometrial ablation are inserted into the uterus through the cervix. Depending on the method chosen, the endometrium is ablated, the instruments are removed, and the patient is allowed to recover for several hours. After the procedure, the patient may feel cramping pain and have a watery or bloody discharge for a few weeks. The results of the procedure are either lighter periods or cessation of menstruation. It is imperative to continue to use some form of contraception due to the increased risk of miscarriage.

Endometrial ablation is not recommended in women with known adenomyosis. According to Pageda et al. (1995), in hysterectomies of women who failed an ablation, 75 percent were found to have adenomyosis. Also, a large study on ablation failures was conducted at the Mayo Clinic in the United States. This study showed that women with adenomyosis had an increased failure risk and required either repeat ablation or hysterectomy (Taran et al., 2013). A study by Riley et al. (2013) showed that 43% of women who failed an endometrial ablation and who went on to have a hysterectomy had adenomyosis. In addition, a study by Beelen et al. (2019) concluded that women with significant period pain had the highest chances of ablation failure.

Dr. Eisen Liang clearly explains why endometrial ablations fail in women with adenomyosis. During an endometrial ablation, about 4 to 9 mm. of tissue is destroyed. For adenomyosis to be diagnosed, the junctional zone must be more that 12 mm. thick. As you can see, the ablation procedure will not destroy even the entire thickness of the junctional zone in women with adenomyosis, so it will not reach the abnormal endometrial tissue within the myometrium. In fact, Dr. Liang states that this procedure will seal off the glands which will result in increased pain after the procedure.

In the Adenomyosis Fighters Support Group, I have noticed that some of the women confuse endometrial ablation with ablation of endometriosis lesions. I think this would be a suitable time to clear up the confusion.

An endometrial ablation burns the inside layer of the uterus (the endometrium). The procedure is done so that the woman will either stop bleeding or have noticeably lighter menstrual bleeding each month. As stated above, this procedure is not recommended if the patient still wants to have children.

Ablation of endometriosis lesions occur outside of the uterus, not within the uterine cavity. This procedure is usually performed through a laparoscopy. Several incisions are made. The incision at the belly button is where the camera will be inserted to view the abdominal organs. Several other small incisions are made where other instruments will be introduced into the abdominal cavity. The surgeon then ablates the endometriosis implants from organs such as the fallopian tubes, the ovaries, the bowel, etc. The reason for this kind of surgery is to reduce the symptoms of endometriosis; however, experts do not recommend this procedure now as endometrial excision is the preferred method of treatment.

In conclusion, an endometrial ablation occurs inside the uterus. Ablation of endometrial implants in the pelvis occurs outside of the uterus. The two surgeries are performed in two separate ways and for completely different reasons. It is extremely important to understand these differences when discussing "ablation."

Estrogen Dominance

"A recent study discovered that some 287 chemicals could be found in the umbilical cord blood of newborns...the average mother has 150 chemicals in her breast milk."

-Marcelle Pick

Five years after my hysterectomy, I learned about estrogen dominance and how it may play a role in the development of adenomyosis. Dr. John Lee was the actual physician who coined the term "estrogen dominance." It refers to a condition where there is insufficient progesterone in relation to estrogen in a woman's body.

The more I learned about estrogen dominance, the more I suspected that I was affected by this hormonal imbalance. This intrigued me, so I went back and pulled out my old medical records to see what my progesterone levels were during the seventeen years that I suffered from adenomyosis and endometriosis. To my surprise, my progesterone levels were never tested. The hormones that were tested were FSH, LH, prolactin, and estradiol.

Estrogen dominance can lead to a whole host of health issues, most notable breast cancer. Pamela Smith (2010) states in her book, *What You Must Know About Women's Hormones*, "If you have PMS, postpartum depression, fibroids or fibrocystic breast disease, there is a good chance that your progesterone-to-estrogen ratio is too low." Today, this abnormal ratio is seen in both endometriosis and adenomyosis. Many times, including in my case, progesterone levels are not tested during regular hormone testing by a family practitioner or gynecologist. This needs to change as progesterone plays such a key role in hormonal balance.

Note: *The following are symptoms associated with estrogen dominance. This is not a comprehensive list*

247

but a list of some of the most common signs of this condition.

- **Allergies, asthma, and sinus congestion**
- **Cold hands and feet**
- **Headaches (including migraines)**
- **Depression and/or anxiety**
- **Breast cancer**
- **Endometrial cancer**
- **Weight gain in the hips, thighs, and abdomen**
- **Fatigue**
- **Insomnia**
- **Foggy thinking**
- **Hypoglycemia**
- **Increased risk of blood clots**
- **Mood swings**
- **Irritability**
- **Osteoporosis**
- **Pre-menopausal bone loss**
- **Polycystic ovarian syndrome**
- **Decreased sex drive**
- **Uterine fibroids**
- **Fibrocystic breast disease**
- **Endometriosis and/or adenomyosis**
- **Premenstrual syndrome**
- **Irregular or heavy periods**
- **Spotting between periods**
- **Infertility**
- **Bloating**
- **Digestive problems**
- **Dry eyes**
- **Unwanted hair growth**
- **Hair loss**
- **Carbohydrate cravings**
- **Magnesium and zinc deficiencies**

As you can see below, the birth control pills that I was prescribed in the earlier years were higher in estrogen and lower in progesterone than those prescribed later in my treatment. In reading my story, my symptoms were better in the later years at a time when I was taking birth control pills that were lower in estrogen and higher in progesterone.

	Estrogen	Progesterone
Ortho Tricyclen®	.035 mg	.18,.215,.25 mg
Ortho Novum 777®	.35 mg	.5, .75, 1 mg
Lo Estrin®	.02 mg	1.0 mg
Yasmin®	.03 mg	3.0 mg

Estrogen and progesterone expression defects have been found in women with adenomyosis. A study by Campo et al. (2012) showed that the overexpression of interleukin 6 (IL-6) in adenomyosis could lead to increased estrogen receptor expression. In addition, they noted that because there is overexpression of cytochrome P450 in women with adenomyosis, overexpression of local estrogen can occur. Also, a defect in progesterone receptor sites was observed. This could explain why so many women with adenomyosis also suffer from estrogen dominance.

We now know that progesterone resistance occurs in both adenomyosis and endometriosis. Progesterone reduces inflammation in the endometrium, and abnormal progesterone signaling can result in inflammation. There are two progesterone receptors in a woman's body – PRA and PRB. PRB has been shown to be hypermethylated in both adenomyosis and endometriosis which leads to progesterone resistance (Wu et al., 2006). Attia et al. (2000) state that PRβ receptor mRNA and protein levels are significantly decreased in endometriotic lesions. Progesterone-related genes have also been shown to be downregulated in endometriosis.

Patel et al. (2017) state, "...progesterone can reversibly inhibit uterine muscle contractility. In effect, labor can be considered a 'progesterone (P4) resistant state...". It should therefore be no surprise that many women who suffer from adenomyosis compare their pain to that of labor. In fact, in my last book, *Adenomyosis: The Women Speak,* some of the women described their pain as follows:

> *"Ten+++++++. Sometimes it gets so bad, all I can do is stay in the fetal position on my bed and swear I am in the final stages of labor."*

> *"Eight to 9 at worst. Labor-like pain during period cramps. I have given birth drug-free, and my cramps are like contractions during early to mid-labor, but without the fabulous "breaks" - It's continuous pain with 'peaks' that are like labor contractions."*

> *"At its worst, I would put it up there with pre-labor. Just longer. I delivered two babies naturally. It felt almost exactly the same before crowning. I couldn't stand for more than a few minutes. Had to drag a stool around so I could make my kids snacks and meals."*

> *"Co-codamol doesn't even come close to touching it. Worse than all 4 of my labours!"*

Many different factors have been proposed as causes of progesterone resistance such as congenital pre-conditioning, chronic inflammation, dioxins (especially TCDD), genetics, mesenchymal stem cell issues, epigenetics, altered microRNA expression, and retinoid resistance. Research is ongoing.

Progestins may help, but some endometriosis patients fail to respond to these medications. However, the progestin dienogest (DNG), aka Visanne®, has been shown in studies to be particularly useful in endometriosis treatment. In fact, one study by Hayashi et al. (2012) showed that dienogest may increase the progesterone receptor B to progesterone receptor A (PRB:PRA) ratio in endometriosis. This same group showed that estrogen receptor β (ERβ) is downregulated by DNG. ERβ is overexpressed in endometriosis, so this downregulation may increase sensitivity to progesterone. Additionally, a study done by Lee et al. (2017) looked at the safety of this progestin when used for more than 12 months in women with an ovarian endometrioma. They found "prolonged daily administration of 2 mg. [dienogest] followed by surgery was associated with a lower recurrence rate of ovarian endometrioma and a reduced pain score and symptoms."

Another interesting study about estrogen expression in adenomyotic tissue was performed in 2014 by Yamanaka et al. This group notes aromatase and estrogen sulphatase levels are higher in adenomyotic tissue. Aromatase is an enzyme that is involved in the conversion of androgens (such as testosterone) to estrogen. Scientists are looking into ways to block aromatase as a way of inhibiting the production of estrogen (see Aromatase Inhibitors for more information).

Yamanaka et al. (2014) states an elevated level of aromatase in adenomyotic tissue suggests a higher sensitivity to estrogen. Also, they note adenomyotic cells appear to be resistant to apoptosis (programmed cell death). The group goes on to say some progestins appear to improve symptoms, so they decided to look at the effects of two progesterone agents in adenomyosis. They found that both endogenous progesterone and DNG increased apoptosis of adenomyotic cells. They concluded both endogenous progesterone and dienogest "directly inhibit cellular stromal cells." The researchers suggest dienogest may be useful in the treatment of adenomyosis.

As you can see, estrogen dominance can be easily missed if the ratio of progesterone to estrogen is not calculated. Hormonal imbalance has largely been underestimated in the past as a cause of gynecological disorders. Today the prevalence of estrogen dominance in the U.S. has been reported to be close to fifty percent. It has been reported that from age 35 to age 50, the level of estrogen in a woman's body will decline by about thirty-five percent while during that same period, the progesterone level will decline by seventy-five percent (Biomedic Labs RX). This explains why estrogen dominance is of utmost concern in older women and probably why, in the past, adenomyosis was reported to predominately affect only older women (we know today that isn't true).

The following is a list of some of the potential causes of estrogen dominance:

- Dysfunction of the adrenal glands
- Anovulation – when a woman does not ovulate, the corpus luteum will not develop. If the corpus luteum is not present, no progesterone will be produced in the second half of the cycle which will lead to an estrogen dominant condition.
- Exposure to xenoestrogens – see Xenoestrogen section.
- Hysterectomy
- Impaired immune system
- Lack of exercise
- Luteal insufficiency – This condition occurs when the corpus luteum does not produce enough progesterone to offset estrogen that is present in a woman's body during the luteal phase of the menstrual cycle. This will lead to an estrogen dominant state. In a study by Prior et al. (1992), out of 18 women with an average age of 29, seven were not ovulating and were not producing progesterone. This condition has been associated with the use of birth control pills.
- Certain medications
- Premenopause and menopause
- Obesity
- Ovarian tumors

- Polycystic ovarian syndrome (PCOS) – This condition occurs when a woman has an excessively elevated level of androgens in her body. When a woman does not ovulate, cysts form on the ovaries. These cysts produce androgens. Although the cause is not known, there has been a link to insulin. Many women with PCOS also have insulin resistance. Symptoms include missed or light periods, infertility, acne, excessive body hair, and weight gain. The disorder can be diagnosed through blood tests that measure hormone levels and by ultrasound. Treatments include medications for diabetes, medications to induce ovulation, birth control pills, a healthy diet, and exercise.
- Poor diet – lack of omega-3 fatty acids, excessive refined carbohydrates, low fiber
- Stress
- Thyroid disorders

The following is a list of some of the possible symptoms of estrogen dominance:

- Adenomyosis
- Allergies
- Anxiety
- Asthma
- Autoimmune disorders such as lupus, Sjogren's disease, and thyroiditis
- Bloating
- Blood clots
- Breast cancer
- Cold hands and feet
- Cravings for carbohydrates
- Decreased sex drive
- Depression
- Digestive problems
- Dry eyes
- Endometrial cancer

- Endometrial polyps
- Endometriosis
- Fatigue
- Fibrocystic breast disease
- Foggy thinking
- Gallbladder issues
- Hair loss
- Headaches, including premenstrual migraines – Estrogen dominance experts Lee and Hopkins (2004) state, "When migraine headaches occur with regularity in women at premenstrual times, they are most likely due to estrogen dominance."
- Heavy menstrual bleeding
- Hypoglycemia
- Infertility
- Irregular menstrual cycles
- Irritability
- Insomnia
- Memory loss
- Mineral deficiencies, especially magnesium and zinc
- Miscarriage
- Mood swings
- Osteoporosis
- Ovarian cysts
- Painful menstrual periods
- Premenopausal bone loss
- Premenstrual syndrome
- Prolonged menstrual bleeding
- Polycystic ovarian syndrome
- Sinus congestion
- Slow metabolism
- Spotting between periods
- Stroke
- Thyroid issues
- Unwanted hair growth
- Uterine cancer
- Uterine fibroids

- Weight gain in the abdomen, hips, and thighs

Excision Surgery

"As twisted as it sounds, I was so happy that I received a diagnosis."

-Bethany Stahl

This type of surgery is done to remove endometriosis, and today, it is considered to be the gold standard treatment for this disorder. The entire endometrial implant is cut out (excised) including the parts that are embedded deep within the affected tissue. This surgery has been shown to be effective at significantly decreasing pain in the long term, and the success of this type of surgery, along with its outperformance of ablation/cauterization, has been documented in many clinical trials.

Ablation of endometrial implants only removes the top, visible part of the lesion, and this leaves residual lesion deep in the tissue which will continue to cause symptoms. According to the Endometriosis Foundation of America, the use of ablation does not work because "this increases the chance of not fully removing the endometriosis lesions and risks damaging the surrounding healthy tissue." They go on to say, "In most cases, ablation/cauterization surgery will not be effective for long-term management of endometriosis because the tissue remains below the surface." I now understand why my laparoscopy failed to relieve my symptoms.

A study by Yeung et al. (2011) showed that the recurrence rate of endometriosis from non-excisional surgery to be between 40 and 60%. This should only clarify why excision surgery has become the gold standard treatment for endometriosis.

According to the Center for Endometriosis Care (2022), "Given the technically difficult, highly advanced surgical skills needed, excision should be performed only in specialized high-volume centers by high-volume surgeons..."

Fibrocystic Breast Disease

"We don't develop courage by being happy every day. We develop it by surviving difficult times and challenging adversity."

-Barbara DeAngelis

Fibrocystic breast disease is the most common type of benign breast disease. Benign breast disease includes non-malignant lesions such as cysts, fibroadenomas, mastalgia, and even nipple discharge.

The symptoms of fibrocystic breast disease usually get worse during PMS and improve once menstruation begins. According to the Mayo Clinic, the symptoms usually affect the upper and outer part of the breast. The cause is still officially unknown, but experts now believe that hormones play a role, especially estrogen.

According to Malherbe et al. (2021), hyperestrogenism is associated with benign breast disease. The researchers state, "the combined use of estrogen and progestin correlated with a 74% risk of benign breast disease. The use of antiestrogens led to a 28% reduction in the prevalence of benign proliferative breast disease." The researchers state that for all palpable lesions in women over 35, mammography with ultrasound examination is needed. Cysts that contain both solid and fluid material need a biopsy. Solid lesions need to have a core biopsy performed to rule out malignancy.

Treatment includes fine needle aspiration or surgical excision for large, painful lumps.

Malherbe et al. (2021) state that the drug metformin may be a treatment for fibrocystic breast disease. Other treatments that may help include NSAIDS, birth control pills, vitamin E, evening primrose oil, use of a heating pad, and use of a firm, supportive bra. Interestingly, studies of the effect of caffeine on this disorder have been inconclusive. Even though it is still recommended to cut down on caffeine to reduce symptoms, the researchers state, "There is no evidence that reducing caffeine improves fibrocystic breast disease or mastalgia." It certainly did not improve symptoms in my case.

Flaxseed

"Fat has become a foul three-letter word in our society We've become a nation of fat phobics, and some of us try to avoid this nutrient at all costs in an effort to lose weight and improve our health. Yet this war on fat has been completely misguided."

-Barry Sears

The actions of flaxseed are thought to be due to the ligan secoisolariciresinol diglucoside (SDG) and alpha-lipoic acid (ALA). Lignans are nonsteroidal phytoestrogens that are metabolized in the liver. They are derived from foods mainly as glucosides, and they produce estrogen-like effects in the body. SDG is broken down into enterolactone and enterodiol, and these substances bind to estrogen receptors which in turn alter cell growth. ALA is a known anti-inflammatory.

Flaxseed has been shown to modulate estrogen metabolism. It also inhibits cell proliferation, angiogenesis, metastasis, and inflammation. All these actions are beneficial for adenomyosis and endometriosis patients. In addition, flaxseed has been shown to inhibit c-Jun n-terminal (pJNK) kinases, mRNAs for B-cell lymphoma gene (Bcl-2), ERα and ERβ, epidermal growth factor (EGF), and insulin-like growth factors. Interestingly, Bcl-2, EGF ERα and ERβ are all increased in adenomyosis and endometriosis.

Flaxseed is an excellent source of omega-3 fatty acids. Fish oil is also an excellent source. Chaudhari et al. (2018) performed a study that looked at the effects of fish oil on endometrial prostaglandin synthesis in the doe. They found that fish oil downregulated the cyclooxygenase 2 pathway (COX-2) which led to decreased endometrial production of the prostaglandins PGF2α and PGE2. PGE2 is a prostaglandin that can cause uterine contractions. PGF2α is activated by oxytocin and can induce labor. This prostaglandin has been found in increased amounts in endometriosis, so this may another reason why so many women with adenomyosis and endometriosis describe their pain as being similar to labor. Since COX-2 and prostaglandins are increased in endometriosis and adenomyosis, this may be part of the reason my symptoms improved when I consumed flaxseed during my ordeal.

This data suggests that the use of flaxseed in adenomyosis and endometriosis may be beneficial.

Gallbladder disease

"It is when I struggle that I strengthen. It is when challenged to my core that I learn the depth of who I am."

-Steve Maraboli

Interestingly, I have seen quite a few comments on the Adenomyosis Fighters Support Group Facebook page from women with adenomyosis who have had gallstones and/or gallbladder surgery. These women wanted to know if there were any connections between gallbladder disease and endometriosis/adenomyosis. Since I also had gallbladder disease and surgery, this piqued my interest, so I did some research.

There are two separate things that might be going on here. First, endometriosis is known to affect areas all over the body. There have been reports of it affecting the gallbladder. Could some of these women have endometriosis of the gallbladder? Possibly.

Another interesting factor that might be at play is that there are estrogen receptors present in the liver. The formation of gallstones is dependent on three things according to Cirillo et al. (2005):

- Supersaturation of biliary cholesterol
- Nucleation of cholesterol monohydrate crystals
- Gallbladder hypomotility

The presence of endogenous estrogen in the liver promotes cholesterol saturation. According to Cirillo et al., "One study found that exogenous estrogens, given either transdermally or orally, affected physiologic markers in a pattern that favored gallstone formation." However, it is also important to note that progestins inhibit gallbladder contraction which is a factor in gallstone formation.

Cirillo et al. (2005) performed a randomized double-blind trial in healthy post-menopausal women from the Women's Health

261

Initiative (WHI) hormone trial and looked at the effect of estrogen and progesterone on gallbladder disease risk. They state that the risk of gallbladder disease was substantially increased by estrogen alone or estrogen plus progesterone. They concluded, "These finding suggest that oral estrogens are causally associated with gallbladder disease, and the magnitude of the effect is not influenced greatly by the presence or absence of progestins."

Other studies have confirmed this association. The Nurse's Health Study in 1974 found that there was an increased risk of cholecystitis (gallbladder disease) in women who took exogenous estrogens, and this risk increased the longer the women took these estrogens. The Atherosclerosis Risk in Communities study group found an increased risk of hospitalization due to gallbladder disease in women who used hormones. Mamandi et al. (2000) found a 1.9 age-adjusted risk factor for cholecystectomy (gallbladder removal) in women who recently started to use estrogen therapy. This same group found an increased risk of appendectomy; however, correlation does not necessarily imply causation. I suffered from a ruptured appendix when I was in college, but my diet was horrible. In addition, my father and brother also had appendicitis, so genetics probably played a role in my case. I have not seen any posts about appendicitis on the Adenomyosis Fighters Support Group Facebook page. This does not necessarily mean that there is no connection. It just means at this point, I have not seen enough evidence yet to suggest a strong connection.

Gonadotropin–Releasing Hormone Agonists (GnRHa)

"Sometimes you will be in control of your illness and other times you'll sink into despair, and that's OK! Freak out, forgive yourself, and try again tomorrow."

-Kelly Hemingway

Although I never took these medications, they can be quite helpful in women with adenomyosis and endometriosis, particularly if the woman wishes to become pregnant.

Gonadotropin-releasing hormone agonists (GNRHa) dramatically reduce estrogen and testosterone levels which will in turn prevent a woman from having a period. This type of medicine will put a woman into temporary menopause, so there will be side effects such as hot flashes and mood swings. Since production of estrogen is prevented during treatment, the adenomyotic tissue will regress since it requires estrogen to grow. However, once the medicine is stopped, the adenomyosis tends to grow back since it will once again be exposed to estrogen.

The use of this medication is limited to three to six months. It can be useful as a pre-treatment to attempted pregnancy. Women who receive GnRHa and immediately try to get pregnant after cessation of GnRHa treatment have greater success than women who are not treated with GnRHa at all.

Some common names of GnRH agonists include Lupron®, Synarel®, Zoladex®, Prostap®, and Enantone®. They can be given either by injection or nasal spray. In addition to hot flashes and mood swings, side effects include insomnia, depression, headaches, low sex drive, acne, and bone thinning.

Hysterectomy

"I don't want my pain and struggle to make me a victim. I want my battle to make me someone's hero."

-unknown

A hysterectomy is the only known cure for adenomyosis. Since the uterus is removed, all adenomyosis will be removed as well. However, a hysterecomy is not a cure for endometriosis.

In a typical laparoscopic hysterectomy, three or four small incisions are made. The incision near the belly button is where the laparoscope will be introduced into the pelvic cavity, and it is used to view the abdominal organs. The other two or three incisions are where the other instruments are introduced into the abdomen to perform the surgery. The uterus/cervix/ovaries/fallopian tubes (what is removed depends on the type of hysterectomy) are removed through one of the small incisions. This surgery results in a quicker recovery for the patient along with less pain as compared to open surgery.

A laparoscopic supracervical hysterectomy (the type that I had) is useful for those with heavy bleeding, fibroids, patients who have a lot of scar tissue, and patients suffering from uterine prolapse. It is not recommended for patients with abnormal Pap smears, those at considerable risk of uterine cancer, or those with a history of cervical or uterine cancer. In this type of hysterectomy, only the uterus is removed.

Before a hysterectomy is performed, gas is introduced into the abdomen to help the surgeon better view the abdominal organs. The gas has a tough time escaping after surgery, so it is common for the patient to feel some shoulder pain especially when sitting up. This soreness will dissipate within a few days.

During a laparoscopic supracervical hysterectomy, some endometrial tissue may remain near the cervical stump. This tissue may continue to bleed monthly resulting in some spotting for the patient. This slight bleeding occurs in about 10% of the women who have this procedure. Sasaki et al. (2014) noticed that in their clinical experience, there was a correlation between cervical stump bleeding and endometriosis. They performed a clinical study in which they looked at the incidence of cervical stump bleeding in 256 patients. 187 patients had no postoperative bleeding, 40 had bleeding within 12 weeks after the operation, and 29 had bleeding after 12 weeks. They found that the patients who bled after 12 weeks were significantly younger and had a higher rate of endometriosis. The group recommends that any patient with a history of endometriosis who prefers to have no further bleeding after hysterectomy should consider a total hysterectomy rather than a supracervical hysterectomy.

DualPortGYN® is a procedure for hysterectomy that was developed by The Center for Innovative GYN Care (CIGC) surgeons. It is one of the safest procedures in the world today.

Dr. Natalya Danilyants (2022) explains how this surgery works through her article, "Groundbreaking Minimally Invasive GYN Surgery" available on CIGC's website. This procedure uses only two incisions – one at the belly button and one very low on the pelvis. It also uses a technique called retroperitoneal dissection which is not used in other hysterectomy procedures. Retroperitoneal dissection allows for better visualization of other structures in the pelvis such as the bowel, bladder, ureters, and uterine artery. Since there is better visualization, the procedure offers an excellent way to avoid injury to these vital structures.

The DualPortGYN® procedure can handle complex procedures such as stage 4 endometriosis or the removal of an exceptionally large uterus that is filled with large fibroids. Of note, this procedure does not use power morcellation. In addition, this procedure uses uterine artery ligation, also known as UAL, which is effective at controlling blood loss. Other hysterectomy procedures do not use UAL. In case adhesions are present, two techniques can be employed during the DualPortGYN® procedure – uterolysis (removal of adhesions from the ureters) and lateral bladder dissection (removal of adhesions affecting the bladder).

Imaging

"Promise me you'll always remember: You're braver than you believe, and stronger than you seem, and smarter than you think."

-A. A. Milne

The two main types of imaging that are used to identify adenomyosis are transvaginal ultrasound (TVS) and magnetic resonance imaging (MRI). Adenomyosis can be picked up by both imaging techniques; however, it is imperative that the sonographer and radiologist are well- trained in adenomyosis detection. According to Dr. Eisen Liang (2021), "...even if an ultrasound is done, which is the first imaging test for uterine conditions, the sonographic features of adenomyosis are rather subtle and can be easily missed."

Endometriosis can sometimes be suspected via TVS. For example, a TVS may be able to pick up the presence of an endometrioma ("chocolate cyst"). A CT can pick up ovarian torsion or cyst rupture that may be due to endometriosis, and an MRI may help in diagnosis. These imaging tests can only raise suspicion of endometriosis, however, and the only way to definitively pick up endometriosis is by laparoscopy.

2D/3D transvaginal ultrasound – This imaging test is performed with a full bladder. The patient lies on her back with her feet in stirrups. The transvaginal probe is covered with a condom and some lubricating gel. The probe is then inserted into the vagina, and images of the reproductive tract are viewed on a computer screen. The technician moves the probe around a bit and takes images of the inside of the uterus, the fallopian tubes, and the ovaries. When finished, the transvaginal probe is removed, and the patient is allowed to urinate.

Adenomyosis can be detected by TVS if the technician/radiologist is knowledgeable regarding adenomyosis as this procedure is highly observer dependent. In a review of adenomyosis by Benagiano et al. (2010), the researchers state, "TVS should be favored as the primary diagnostic tool, although substantial experience and specific training is required to make sonography a useful diagnostic tool." According to Streuli et al. (2014), red flags include "globular uterus, asymmetry of uterine walls, poorly defined junctional zone, poorly defined focus of abnormal myometrial echotexture, distorted and heterogeneous myometrial echotexture, myometrial linear striations and myometrial cysts." Although possible to diagnose this disorder by TVS, it will remain difficult to do so until one specific set of criteria is adopted by the medical community. It needs to be noted that Exacoustos et al. (2011) report the presence of myometrial cysts on a 2D TVS can indicate adenomyosis with an accuracy of 78 percent and a specificity of 98 percent. In addition, this same group of researchers state adenomyosis can be detected on a 3D TVS with an accuracy of 85 percent if the junctional zone (JZ) difference in thickness in > 4mm. throughout the uterine wall.

In doing research for this book, I was comforted to know that Dr. Camran Nezhat of the Nezhat Institute in California recognizes that a transvaginal ultrasound may be painful for women with endometriosis. He states that he works with women to minimize and pain and discomfort while performing the test. I hope that more gynecological physicians/sonographers realize this in the future.

Magnetic resonance imaging (MRI) - This imaging technique has become extremely valuable for adenomyosis diagnosis. On T-2 weighted magnetic resonance images, the junctional zone can be visualized quite well. On MRI, there are three distinct zones that can be identified in the uterine wall. The endometrium has a high signal intensity. Underneath this layer is an area of low signal intensity which is the JZ. The myometrium has a medium signal intensity. When bleeding occurs in the adenomyotic tissue, the signal intensity may become high.

A normal JZ is about 4 to 9 mm. wide, and the widening of this area to 12 mm. or more is highly suggestive of adenomyosis. MRI has recently been found to be the most useful test for detecting adenomyosis when fibroids or other abnormalities are also present. According to Novellas et al. (2011), the presence of microcysts within the JZ or myometrium are indicative of adenomyosis. These cysts can vary from 2 to 7 mm. in diameter. However, according to this same group, these cysts can only be detected in about fifty percent of cases. An adenomyoma is easier to detect, but it must be differentiated from a uterine fibroid. A fibroid can be differentiated from an adenomyoma by looking at its border. A fibroid has a distinct border whereas an adenomyoma bleeds into the surrounding myometrium leaving a fuzzy border.

Dueholm et al. (2001) state that the use of both TVS and MRI gives the most accurate results in the diagnosis of adenomyosis. However, diagnosis through MRI is by far not an absolute. Dr. Albee at the Center for Endometriosis Care (2016) states, "I am not hopeful that we will soon be able to rely on it to diagnose the isolated, scattered areas of glands lost among the muscle cells because of their small size."

Since I suffered from adenomyosis from 1990-2007, an MRI was never ordered in my case. Information about the thickening of the junctional zone was not widely available to physicians at that time. The new knowledge about the junctional zone should prompt more physicians to order an MRI if adenomyosis is suspected. In addition, insurance companies need to be aware of this and not reject coverage of an MRI in a woman with suspected adenomyosis.

Infertility

"The clock is definitely ticking, as we know millions of women still live awash in anguish, just as they did thousands of years ago and just as they will centuries from now unless we steer ourselves faster toward the long-elusive cure. Four thousand years is long enough: the time has come to end the empire of endometriosis."

-Drs. Camran, Farr, and Ceana Nezhat

Women with adenomyosis and endometriosis are known to have problems with infertility.

In animal experiments, baboons with adenomyosis have had infertility problems and endometriosis (Campo et al., 2012). According to Garavaglia et al. (2015), "The more and more frequent diagnosis in fertility clinics during the diagnostic work-up and its detection in baboons with lifelong infertility have suggested that [adenomyosis] may develop in young women and may have important consequences on fertility."

Factors that may interfere with fertility in adenomyosis include:

- Painful sex
- Adhesions
- Increased oxidative stress within the uterus
- Hostile uterine environment
- Other endocrine disorders may be present such as luteal phase issues, ovulatory disorders, and luteinized unruptured follicle syndrome.

**Source is from Sinervo et al. (2016)

DeSouza et al. (1995) report in women with painful and heavy periods who also had problems with infertility had a 54% incidence of JZ hyperplasia. Seventy percent of these women never had children. Studies have also shown an increase in the risk of pre-term delivery in women with both adenomyosis and endometriosis. In adenomyosis, this could possibly be due to failure of deep implantation of the placenta due to JZ thickening. In fact, in women with adenomyosis, placental abruption has been reported (Harada et al., 2019).

In adenomyosis, it has been shown that the uterus may contain an excessive amount of free radicals, and this may damage the fertilized egg (Campo et al., 2012). According to Garavaglia et al. (2015), "the presence of high levels of intrauterine free radicals has a negative influence during sperm transport, implantation and pregnancy." Ota et al. (1998) studied the levels of nitric oxide in the endometrium of women with adenomyosis and endometriosis and found that the level of nitric oxide was significantly higher in these women than in the control group. Elevated levels of nitric oxide have been shown to reduce sperm motility and increase uterine peristalsis. Both factors could play a role in infertility.

The increase in uterine contractions (hyperperistalsis) seen in adenomyosis could possibly affect sperm transport and proper implantation of the embryo. In addition, the increased contractions may cause pre-term delivery and premature rupture of membranes. Since prostaglandins are overproduced in adenomyosis, and prostaglandins are involved in dilation and thinning of the cervix, an increase in prostaglandins could explain why pregnancies may not be able to be maintained in some women with adenomyosis.

In one study regarding endometriosis, the chances of conceiving without any surgical intervention were as follows:

Stage I and II – 60%
Stage III – 15-20%
Stage IV – none in this study, but it is generally accepted that a small percentage may conceive (around 5%)

After surgical excision of endometriosis:

Stage I and II – 80 to 85%
Stage III – 70 to 75%
Stage IV – 50 to 60%

**Source is from Sinervo et al. (2016)

According to Bulletti et al. (2010), "Infertile women are 6-8 times more likely to have endometriosis than fertile women."

Possible reasons for infertility in endometriosis include the following:

1. Distorted anatomy in the pelvis caused by adhesions
2. Hormonal dysregulation
3. Ovulatory abnormalities
4. Endocrine dysfunction including luteal phase defects and impaired folliculogenesis
5. Excess peritoneal fluid with "high concentration of activated macrophages, prostaglandins, IL-1, TNF, and proteases" which can adversely affect "function of the oocyte, sperm, embryo, or fallopian tube." (Bulletti et al., 2010)
6. Increase in uterine contractions which may lead to failure of implantation.

If both endometriosis and adenomyosis are present, the chances of implantation may even be lower due to the increased uterine contractions and JZ hyperplasia.

In Vitro Fertilization

"It is not easy to talk about a condition once dismissed as 'the career woman's disease'. But women will continue to suffer until we realize the cost of ignoring it."

-Hilary Mantel

Sadly, it is now known that in vitro fertilization success rates in adenomyosis patients are low. Dr. Keith Isaacson (2019) states that "...patients with adenomyosis actually have lower implantation rates after undergoing IVF. They have lower clinical pregnancy rates if they're undergoing IVF, and they have lower live birth rates...It is actually a 41% decrease in the live birth rate."

Salim et al. (2012) evaluated 275 women who underwent in vitro fertilization/intracytoplasmic sperm injection (IVF/ICSI) for the first time. Two hundred fifty-six of these women did not have adenomyosis (control group) and 19 women were confirmed to have adenomyosis via transvaginal ultrasound. They found that the clinical pregnancy rate was 22.2% in women with adenomyosis compared to 47.2% in those without the disorder. The ongoing pregnancy rate was 11.1% in women with adenomyosis and 45.9% in women without the disorder. In addition, the miscarriage rate was 50.0% in women with adenomyosis compared to 2.8% in the control group. This study clearly shows that adenomyosis has a significant negative impact on women who undergo IVF/ICSI due to infertility.

In 2012, Vercellini et al. (2014) published a meta-analysis and found that "women with adenomyosis had a 28% reduction in the likelihood of clinical pregnancy at IVF/ICSI compared with women without adenomyosis." In this study, the researchers found that 31.9% of the women with adenomyosis suffered a miscarriage while only 14.1% of those without adenomyosis suffered a miscarriage.

Campo et al. (2012) state that in women who undergo IVF, evaluation of the junctional zone thickness via MRI is the best way to predict implantation failure. This group also noted that if the patient had a JZ thickness of 10 mm. or more, treatment with a GnRH analog prior to IVF had an improvement in the success rate of the procedure. GnRHa decreases the expression of aromatase which is overexpressed in women with adenomyosis.

Interestingly, Tremellen & Russell (2011) looked at 4 women with adenomyosis who had undergone failed IVF attempts due to failure of implantation of good embryos and found that a "prominent aggregation of macrophages within the superficial endometrial glands" possibly interfered with embryo implantation. See Platelet Aggregation for more information.

Kuivasaari et al. (2005) compared IVF/ISCI outcomes between stage I/II endometriosis patients, stage III/IV endometriosis patients, and patients with infertility due to tubal problems (control). They were able to show that the pregnancy rate was significantly lower in women with stage III/IV disease compared to the other two groups. This shows that the worse the endometriosis, the lower the rate of a successful IVF/ICSI procedure.

Pop-Trajkovic et al. (2013) performed a similar study. They also found that stage III/IV endometriosis conferred a worse prognosis for a successful IVF outcome.

Irritable Bowel Syndrome

"Ruling out IBS can be difficult for non-specialists, especially since IBS can flare during menstruation, which may be one of the main reasons why so many women with bowel endometriosis are incorrectly diagnosed with IBS."

-Dr. Camran Nezhat

According to Saidi et al. (2020), those with endometriosis are two to three times more likely to be diagnosed with IBS. According to Lee et al. (2018), 52% of patients with endometriosis had a diagnosis of IBS. This shows how often endometriosis can be misdiagnosed as IBS.

Symptoms of IBS include:

- Alternating constipation and diarrhea
- Abdominal pain that is relieved by bowel movements
- Significant bloating
- Nausea

At the Center for Endometriosis Care, Dr Ken Sinervo (2022) states that over 20 percent of their patients report constipation. This could be due to narrowing or kinking of the bowel, adhesions, and/or inflammatory mediators that can alter motility of the intestine. Diarrhea is seen in about 2/3 of patients with endometriosis. Dr. Sinervo also states that "in patients with invasive and obstructive endometriosis, they often have a combination of constipation followed by diarrhea." Note that these are the same symptoms that occur in IBS. According to Dr. Sinervo, adhesions and/or narrowing of the bowel by endometriosis can cause severe constipation, and when the hard stool above the endometriosis lesion is passed, patients will often have reflex diarrhea afterwards.

As far as treatment, Dr. Sinervo states that many patients may respond to pharmaceutical treatments such as birth control, aromatase inhibitors, GnRH agonists, and progestins, but they may ultimately need surgical intervention. It is important to go to a physician who is an expert in bowel endometriosis, such as Dr. Sinervo, to get the best care; otherwise, the patient may end up with either incomplete treatment or no treatment at all. In addition, Dr. Sinervo (2022) states that it is important to evaluate the entire bowel because "as much as 10% [of invasive endometriosis] lies outside the pelvis or concurrently with rectosigmoid endometriosis."

Dr. Camran Nezhat (2021) explained the differences between IBS and bowel endometriosis. He states that in IBS, pain is moderate while in bowel endometriosis, the pain is severe. He also states that in IBS, upper abdominal pain is more common while in bowel endometriosis, lower abdominal pain is much more common. Also, in bowel endometriosis, extreme pain during bowel movements occurs much more often. All of these should have been red flags in my case; however, my doctors were not well versed in endometriosis and/or adenomyosis, so the diagnosis was missed.

Although issues such as gluten and lactose intolerance or small intestinal bacterial overgrowth (SIBO) may contribute to these bowel problems, Dr. Sinervo also believes that another factor may be at play. According to Dr. Sinervo (2022), "In patients with endometriosis (and possible adenomyosis), there is a massive increase in the release of inflammatory mediators, which can be seen in the fluid surrounding the bowel...the bowel becomes irritated and those inflammatory mediators...slow or alter the motility [of the intestine]. Patients often have a decreased appetite because of this, and in extreme cases, even acid reflux symptoms."

Moore et al. (2017) found that in these cases, a low FODMAP diet may help. FODMAP stands for fermentable oligosaccharides, disaccharides, monosaccharides, and polyols. These are the types of foods that may play a role in IBS. The

FODMAP diet is a temporary diet in which foods in the above listed categories are eliminated and then added back in to see which ones cause symptoms. Since this kind of diet eliminates a lot of foods, it should only be undertaken while working closely with a doctor. According to Dr. Hazel Veloso (2022), the elimination part of the diet should only be followed for two to six weeks.

Examples of high FODMAP foods includes:

- Dairy products such as cream, ice cream and yogurt
- Products containing wheat including barley, rye, and couscous
- Beans and peas such as chickpeas, kidney beans, and black-eyed peas
- Some vegetables including cauliflower, celery, garlic, onions, and mushrooms
- Some fruits including cherries, grapefruit, mango, plums, and prunes
- Soy milk and soybeans
- Molasses and high fructose corn syrup
-

Examples of low FODMAP foods include:

- Some cheeses such as brie, cheddar, and feta
- Some grains such as oats and brown rice
- Almond milk
- Some vegetables such as potatoes, tomatoes, cucumbers, broccoli, carrots, and kale
- Some fruits such as pineapple, grapes, oranges, strawberries, bananas, lemons, and limes
- Maple syrup and powdered sugar
- Nuts such as almonds, peanuts, pecans, and walnuts
- Meats such as beef, chicken, pork
- Eggs

Dr. Hazel Veloso (2022) states that a low FODMAP diet reduces symptoms in 86% of people with IBS.

In addition to the low FODMAP diet, following an anti-inflammatory or gluten-free diet may help. Other helpful ideas include physical therapy, eating smaller and more frequent meals, use of probiotics, and lowering salt intake.

Leiomyomas (Uterine Fibroids)

"If opening your eyes, or getting out of bed, or holding a spoon, or combing your hair is the daunting Mount Everest you climb today, that is okay."

-Carmen Ambrosio

Leiomyomas, also known as uterine fibroids, are growths that originate from the myometrium. They are the most common uterine disorder and affect up to 80 percent of all women. There are several types of fibroids depending on their location within the uterus and include pedunculated, subserous, submucous, intramural and intracavity. For unknown reasons, African American women are two to three times more likely to suffer from fibroids compared to other races.

Symptoms of leiomyomas include heavy bleeding that can lead to anemia, pelvic pain, pressure on the bladder, and painful bowel movements. In addition, fibroids may interfere with fertility. To this day, it is often difficult to distinguish a fibroid from an adenomyoma.

Pelvic exams are not the best way to diagnose the presence of fibroids in the uterus. The best way to detect fibroids is through an ultrasound.

Pharmaceutical treatments include birth control pills which reduce estrogen levels. Surgical treatment includes a myomectomy (which preserves the uterus if future fertility is desired) or a hysterectomy. Uterine fibroid embolization is another option although fertility may be compromised after this procedure.

Since fibroids depend on estrogen to grow, they may shrink after menopause. However, according to CIGC (2022), "Fibroids can also undergo 'degeneration' after menopause and loss of blood supply. Calcific degeneration...calcifies the fibroids, turning

279

them into extremely hard masses that are difficult to remove." They go on to state that these calcified masses can cause discomfort.

A specialized myomectomy surgery developed by CIGC is now available. This procedure is called the Laparoscopically Assisted Abdominal Myomectomy (LAAM®). Dr. Paul Mackoul explains how this surgery is done in his article, "Advanced Fibroid Removal with the LAAM® Myomectomy" available on CIGC's website. It is a combination of a laparoscopy and a mini laparotomy. Only two incisions are needed – one at the belly button, and the other slightly larger incision low on the pelvis. A tourniquet is put in place at the lower incision to control blood loss. The fibroids are removed through that lower incision. After the removal of each fibroid, the uterus is stitched up using the standard suturing method. These sutures are stronger than those used during a robotic surgery or a laparoscopy. The most interesting part of this procedure is that the physician can feel the uterus as he/she works. This means that even small fibroids or fibroids that are not visible during laparoscopy can be "felt" and removed. This ensures that all fibroids are removed – something that cannot be done during a laparoscopy or a robotic procedure.

LAAM® is a safe procedure with better control of blood loss and the ability to identify all fibroids present in the uterus. Power morcellation is never used, and recovery time is much shorter than a regular myomectomy.

It is important to note, however, that this procedure should only be performed on women who desire pregnancy. The physicians at CIGC state that if a patient does not desire pregnancy, she should strongly consider a partial hysterectomy instead of the LAAM® procedure. In addition, they also say that a uterine artery embolization (UAE) is not advisable for women who wish to become pregnant in the future. A UAE does not remove the fibroid – it merely shrinks it. They state, "Fibroids present deep in the uterus and near the uterine cavity can still cause problems with fertility after UAE simply because the embryo may implant near the fibroid resulting in miscarriage."

Mirena®

"We must accept finite disappointment, but never lose infinite hope."

-Martin Luther King, Jr.

The Mirena® is a small T-shaped intrauterine device that delivers a small amount of a progestin over the course of five years. Each arm is about 3.2 cm. long, and the body that contains the progestin is about 3.2 cm. long. It is used to control heavy menstrual bleeding and can be inserted in a doctor's office.

The process of insertion is fairly simple. The patient lies on her back with her feet in stirrups. Prior to the insertion of the IUD, the physician will do a manual exam to assess proper placement. First, a speculum is used to open the vagina, and a tenaculum is inserted to hold the cervix in place. The physician then used a sound to determine the length of the uterus. This will help in the placement of the IUD. It is then inserted and opens into a T-shape once in place. It only takes a couple of minutes to insert. Some women report pinching or cramping during the procedure, but this is usually minor pain and should dissipate quickly. A couple of strings hang down into the vagina after placement, and the patient is advised to check these strings often to ensure that the IUD is still in place.

This device is useful in treating women with endometriosis. However, the use of this product is a little more complicated in women who suffer from adenomyosis. A study by Lee et al. (2016) found that the use of Mirena in women with adenomyosis was less effective than in other women. In women with a uterus larger than 150 ml., the patient was more likely to discontinue use. In women with a uterus larger than 314 ml., the discontinuation rate was 70%. In addition, in women whose uterus is distorted from adenomyosis and/or fibroids, the Mirena may be expelled from the body.

If an adenomyosis patient can tolerate the Mirena®, it may help her. In a study by Cho et al. (2008), this type of IUD was found to significantly reduce pain and bleeding in adenomyosis patients, and the reduction of symptoms continued for 36 months. Sheng et al. (2009) was able to obtain comparable results in their study and showed that cancer antigen 125 (CA125) levels dramatically dropped in these women (CA125 levels have been shown to be high in both adenomyosis and endometriosis). Mansukhani et al. (2013) report almost 50 percent of the women were asymptomatic after six months of treatment with a satisfaction rate of 80 percent. Yet another study by Fong and Singh (1999) showed the successful treatment of a grossly enlarged uterus due to adenomyosis using this system. Fong and Singh also noted a marked decrease in uterine size at 12 months and reported the resolution of pain and bleeding in this patient.

Platelet Aggregation and Mean Platelet Volume (MPV)

"As in endometriosis, adenomyotic lesions show significantly increased platelet aggregation..."

-Liu et al (2016)

This is an extremely complicated topic, but it is necessary to touch on it with a basic explanation since platelet aggregation has been shown to be a part of both adenomyosis and endometriosis. Additionally, at one point I had a high MPV value in my bloodwork which might have indicated platelet aggregation during the time that I suffered with symptoms of both disorders.

Let's start with some basic information.

Platelets, also known as thrombocytes, are made in the bone marrow and are involved in blood clotting. If a blood vessel is damaged, platelets come to the site of damage and form a clot, also known as a thrombus. They stick together through a process called adhesion. As other platelets come to the site, they pile on top of each other in a process called aggregation.

Mean platelet volume (MPV) refers to the size and activity of the platelets. The higher the MPV, the larger the platelet size. Larger platelets produce large amounts of cellular mediators such cytokines and chemokines. These substances promote inflammation. Another cellular mediator that is produced by platelets is thromboxane. Thromboxane may be involved in vasoconstriction and may lead to uterine cramps.

It is known that the endometrium goes through a process of tissue injury and repair, also known as TIAR, each month during menstruation. TIAR can also be caused by any kind of trauma at the junctional zone in the uterus. Examples include birth, C-section, dilation and curettage (D&C), and chronic uterine hyperperistalsis (excessive uterine contractions). During this process of TIAR, macrophages, a type of white blood cell that is also known as a leukocyte, interact with activated platelets which leads to cytokine secretion from both cell types.

During the TIAR process, platelets induce a process called epithelial to mesenchymal transition (EMT) and fibroblast to myofibroblast transdifferentiation (FMT).

EMT is a process in which epithelial cells are transformed into mesenchymal cells. Epithelial cells are polarized and form strong cell-to-cell bonds. Mesenchymal cells do not have these strong bonds, and they can migrate and differentiate into other types of cells. Mesenchymal cells are also resistant to apoptosis (programmed cell death) and have an increase in extracellular matrix (ECM) products. When epithelial cells transform into mesenchymal cells, levels of e-cadherin decrease, and levels of matrix metalloproteinases increase.

There are three types of EMTs. Type 2 EMT is the process we are concerned with in this discussion. Type 2 EMT resolves once inflammation is gone; however, fibrosis (an increase in fibrous tissue) can occur with chronic inflammation. Fibrosis can cause scarring and hardening of tissue and is due to excess extracellular matrix (ECM) products.

Now, if you followed all of that, let's get to how all of this is involved in adenomyosis and endometriosis.

A study by Bodur et al. (2015) found that MPV and platelet distribution width (PDW) were significantly higher in adenomyosis patients compared to a control group. In fact, they found that" women with adenomyosis were five times more likely to have elevated MPV values." They also stated that a higher MPV value "may correspond to the increased number of both platelet-leukocyte and platelet-platelet aggregates." The group concluded gynecologists should "...give priority on adenomyosis when premenopausal parous patient with a history of curettages admitted with a complaint of dysmenorrhea and elevated levels of MPV."

Liu et al. (2016) took a close look at the platelet aggregation process in women with adenomyosis. They stated, "...platelets play critical roles in the development of adenomyosis by promoting proliferation, angiogenesis, increasing ECM deposits, and [smooth muscle metaplasia], resulting in fibrosis. Platelets may also be involved in uterine hyperactivity and myometrial hyperinnervation." According to the researchers, activated platelets induce the activation of transforming growth factor β1 (TGF-β1)/Smad signaling pathway which leads to both EMT and FMT. This further leads to the increase of invasive and migratory capability of cells. The entire process leads to smooth muscle metaplasia (SMM) and fibrosis. In adenomyosis patients, the group found (compared to controls) significantly higher levels of platelet aggregation, microvessel density (MVD), immunoreactivity to vascular endothelial growth factor (VEGF), proliferating cell nuclear antigen (PCNA), transforming growth factor beta 1 (TGF-β1), p-Smad3, vimentin, alpha smooth muscle actin (α-SMA), collagen 1, and lipoxygenase (LOX). The immunoreactivity to e-cadherin and PRB was significantly reduced. As stated previously, e-cadherin is decreased during EMT. The increased staining of α-SMA in adenomyotic lesions suggest FMT because α-SMA is a marker for myofibroblasts. In addition, Kalluri & Weinberg (2009) state that α-SMA and collagen I are markers that "characterize the mesenchymal products generated by EMTs that occur during the development of fibrosis..."

Liu et al (2016) pointed out two very interesting things in their study. First, uterine size may indicate the severity of disease. They state, "Our finding that uterus size in women with adenomyosis correlated positively with the staining levels of α-SMA, collagen I and the extent of fibrosis seems to suggest that the uterus size is directly proportional to the extent of progression of adenomyosis." Second, thromboxane, released from activated platelets, may promote severe uterine cramping. They state, "...the release of [thromboxane A2] by activated platelets may likely promote uterine hyperperistalsis or even dysperistalsis, as documented in adenomyosis."

One last important observation has to do with elevated levels of prolactin that has noted in adenomyosis. Hyperprolactinemia has been shown to occur in adenomyosis, and interestingly, prolactin is a strong cofactor for platelet aggregation.

Zhu et al (2016) was able to show that anti-platelet treatments "dose-dependently suppressed myometrial infiltration, improved generalized hyperalgesia, reduced uterine contractility, and lowered plasma corticosterone levels, improved the expression of some proteins known to be involve in adenomyosis and slowed down the process of fibrinogenesis."

In conclusion, increased platelet aggregation is increased in endometriosis and adenomyosis. MPV may be elevated in these patients, and physicians should keep an eye on this blood test when there is suspicion for these disorders.

Progesterone, Vitamin D, and Bone Health

"Some days are better, some days are worse. Look for the blessing instead of the curse. Be positive, stay strong, and get enough rest. You can't do it all, but you can do your best."

-Doe Zantamata

Recent studies have shown that progesterone helps to promote new bone growth by stimulating osteoblast differentiation. An osteoblast is a cell that makes bone. Low progesterone levels have been linked to lower levels of osteoblasts that are needed to rebuild bone. As a result, low progesterone levels may lead to bones that are weak and brittle. It is reported that progesterone stimulates new bone formation while estradiol inhibits bone resorption. Molecular studies using polymerase chain reaction (PCR) have shown that progesterone has action in bone formation. According to a study by MacNamara, O'Shaughnessy, Manduca, and Loughrey (1995), "The finding that [progesterone] is expressed at both the level of [messenger RNA] and protein in several osteoblast-like cell lines as well as in human primary osteoblast cultures indicates that bone-forming osteoblast cells are direct targets for progesterone action."

According to Dr. John Lee, M.D. (2012), after treating his patients with a transdermal progesterone cream for three years, he identified a 15% improvement in bone mineral density even though there was no estrogen supplementation. Seifert-Klauss and Prior (2010), reported that progesterone and anti-resorptive drugs in combination increase bone mineral density and increase bone formation.

In a more recent study by Seifert-Klauss (2012), the researchers state, "Data from a pilot study in perimenopausal women also suggested that higher progesterone levels, as seen in the luteal phase of ovulatory cycles, may be associated with more bone formation and with slightly less bone resorption than anovulatory cycles in which progesterone levels are low (<5.8 ng/ml)." This led a large 2-year prospective observational study called PENKO. Data from this study has shown that women who do not ovulate regularly have an increased risk of loss of bone mineral density.

Since progesterone appears to play a critical role in bone health, I became very suspicious that the cause of my failed spinal fusions may be linked to estrogen dominance and progesterone resistance that has been documented in both endometriosis and adenomyosis. According to Seifert-Klauss and Prior (2012), "Subclinical ovulatory disturbances may pose a risk for bone remodeling imbalance and bone loss despite regular, estrogen-sufficient menstrual cycles." In my case, I did have regular 28-day cycles. In addition, during the few times I had my hormones tested over my 17-year ordeal, my estrogen levels always came back normal. Also, according to Seifert-Klauss and Prior (2010), "The fact that bone morphogenic protein play a crucial role in both ovulation and bone metabolism points towards a functional link between bone and reproductive systems...." It is interesting to note that in my case, the third fusion finally succeeded with the use of synthetic bone morphogenic protein during surgery.

Vitamin D levels in endometriosis tend to be lower than in women without the disease; however, technically, no consensus exists about the relationship of low vitamin D levels and endometriosis in the scientific community.

A study done by Ciavattini et al. (2016) looked at the levels of vitamin D in 49 women with a single ovarian endometrioma. Out of the 49 patients, 42 of them were found to have low vitamin D levels. Oiu et al. (2020) evaluated nine studies regarding vitamin D and endometriosis and concluded that low vitamin D levels were a risk factor for endometriosis. They found that women with endometriosis who had never used hormones had lower vitamin D levels as compared to controls. In addition, they found a negative correlation between disease severity and vitamin D levels. This means that the lower the vitamin D levels, the more severe the disease and vice versa.

Mehdizadehkashi et al. (2021) looked at the effect of vitamin D supplementation in patients with endometriosis. This was a randomized, double-blind, placebo-controlled trial. They found that vitamin D supplementation significantly decreased pain levels in women with endometriosis. Additionally, they showed that C-reactive protein (CRP), a marker of inflammation, significantly reduced, and total antioxidant capacity (TAC) increased when compared to placebo. They concluded, "...our study demonstrated that vitamin D intake in patients with endometriosis resulted in a significant improvement of pelvic pain, total-/HDL-cholesterol ratio, hs-CRP, and TAC levels, but did not affect other clinical symptoms and metabolic profiles."

Dr. Ken Sinervo (2021) discussed the role of small intestinal bacterial overgrowth (SIBO) in the role of weak bones. SIBO is a condition where there is overgrowth of certain bacteria in the small intestine, some of which are not normally seen in that area of the GI tract. SIBO can occur in any condition where the transit of food is slowed. Some of these conditions include Crohn's disease, celiac disease, and diabetes. It is also commonly seen after surgery. If endometriosis has caused distortion or obstruction of the bowel, SIBO may result. SIBO is also known to reduce calcium absorption which may result in weak bones. Many patients with endometriosis also suffer from IBS, so these patients may also have SIBO. One antibiotic, Xifaxin, is effective in treating SIBO although it is expensive.

Ghosal and Srivastava (2014) looked at many different studies on the relationship between IBS and SIBO and found that the occurrence of SIBO varied from 4 to 78% in IBS patients. The frequency of SIBO among controls varied from 1 to 40%. They found that a glucose hydrogen breath test (GHBT) had "a low sensitivity to diagnose SIBO."

Several years later, in 2020, Ghoshal et al. performed a meta-analysis on SIBO in patients with different types of IBS. They found that 36.7% of IBS patients also had SIBO. They also found that patients with GHBT positive SIBO were more likely to have diarrhea-predominant IBS.

Considering my abnormal Pg/E2 ratio, infertility issues, adenomyosis and endometriosis diagnoses, and failed spinal fusions, it appears to me that estrogen dominance and progesterone resistance may have played a critical role in my failed spinal fusions. It is important for endometriosis and adenomyosis patient to be aware of this connection between low progesterone and bone health, following up quickly with their physicians if any bone-related issues show up.

Rectovaginal endometriosis

Rectovaginal endometriosis (RVE) refers to endometriosis that is present in the space between the vagina and the bowel. This area is referred to as the cul-de-sac or the Pouch of Douglas. Endometriosis that is present in this location can cause severe pain, intestinal problems (including intestinal obstruction), bloating, dyschezia (painful bowel movements) and dyspareunia (painful intercourse).

According to Kruse et al. (2012), "Infiltrating endometriosis is defined as the localization of endometriotic tissue more than 5 mm. below the peritoneal surface. Rectovaginal endometriosis (RVE) comprises infiltrating lesions of the rectovaginal septum with variable involvement of the vagina, rectum, and uterosacral ligaments."

According to Dr. Tamer Seckin of the Endometriosis Foundation of America (2020), "...when the patient comes to the office, you check the patient, there's tenderness in the cul-de-sac on one side. Even though they do not have any advanced endometriosis that we can really tell most of the time by sonogram, called endometrioma or rectovaginal disease by exam, we can suspect by tenderness, it is most likely endometriosis." He goes on to explain that in his practice, about 70% of cases where they excised endometriosis, the lesions were on the bowel and in the cul-de-sac region.

Dr. Camran Nezhat (2021) explains that when endometriosis has impacted the bowel, "the most common findings during a pelvic exam include the presence of painful nodules and/or tenderness in the rectovaginal cul-de-sac (Pouch of Douglas), and on the uterosacral ligaments. Vaginal and uterine pain may also be

"

present." He goes on to explain that an obliterated cul-de-sac may be felt by doing a bi-digital exam. He points out that studies have shown that in women with an obliterated cul-de-sac, bowel endometriosis is three times more likely to be present.

Studies have shown that TVS may be useful in the diagnosis of RVE; however, it will not pick up endometrial implants above the rectosigmoid junction. Also, the use of saline solution or water contrast in the vagina and rectum, respectively, improves the ability to obtain a correct diagnosis of RVE. The problem is that special training is needed to properly perform these tests.

Dr. Camran Nezhat (2021) explains that in cases of bowel endometriosis, he has found that TVS, transrectal ultrasound, and double contrast barium enema are the most useful tests. He states that one study found that TVS had a sensitivity of 91 percent and a specificity of 98%. However, other studies have shown less promising results. As others have stated, he says that the value of the test is dependent on the experience of the sonographer and radiologist. The transrectal ultrasound also has its limitations as it cannot view anything past the rectosigmoid junction. The reliability of this ultrasound is around the same for TVS, and again, accurate results are dependent on the experience of those reading and interpreting the results. MRI can be useful as it can view parts of the colon that regular ultrasounds cannot.

Kruse et al. (2012) state that birth control pills, levonorgestrel-releasing IUD, and progestins can all be effective treatments for rectovaginal endometriosis.

GnRH agonists can help to reduce the lesion size and to reduce pain; however, these medications can only be used short-term, and the lesions/pain will return once the medication is stopped. A study by Vercellini et al. (2005) showed that treatment of RVE with either a birth control pill or a progestin reduced pain, painful intercourse, and dyschezia significantly after 12 months of treatment. Fedele et al. (2001) tested the use of the levonorgestrel-releasing IUD in 11 patients with RVE, and they found that pain decreased rather quickly (three to six months), but the reduction in painful intercourse symptoms took longer. Aromatase inhibitors have been shown to decrease symptoms of pain and painful intercourse; however, symptoms recur after treatment. Remorgida et al. (2007) observed 12 women with RVE over a 6-month period who used the aromatase inhibitor letrozole along with norethisterone. They noted a significant decrease in pain and painful intercourse in the first month, but the pain returned to baseline levels after 6 months of treatment.

The surgical treatment of RVE is complicated and may need a multi-disciplinary approach to be successful. Kruse et al. (2012) describe three different surgeries that can be performed depending on the depth of invasion into the bowel wall – shaving, discoid excision, and rectal resection. See the section on Colorectal Resection for more information.

Uterine Artery Embolization (UAE)

"Start by doing what's necessary; then do what's possible; and suddenly you are doing the impossible."

-St. Francis of Assisi

Also known as UAE, uterine artery embolization cuts off blood supply to parts of the uterus. This results in tissue death and scarring of the uterine tissue. This procedure has been used for many years in treating uterine fibroids.

Dr. Eisen Liang and Dr. Bevan Brown (2021) of the Sydney Fibroid Clinic in Sydney, Australia found that many of the women they treated using this procedure for fibroids also had adenomyosis or that adenomyosis had been mistaken for fibroids. They were able to determine in their study that UAE was 90% effective at treating adenomyosis.

During the UAE procedure, which is performed by an interventional radiologist, a small incision is made in the top of the leg near the groin. A guidewire and catheter are inserted in the femoral artery, and they are threaded up into the uterine artery. Particles are injected until the artery is blocked. The guidewire and catheter are removed, and the incision is sealed. The patient must lie flat for the next couple of hours.

Dr. Eisen Liang (2021) explains how UAE can be effective for women with adenomyosis in his book, *Could it be Adenomyosis? The (Bad) Cousin of Endometriosis*. Small particles are injected into the uterine arteries which causes death of adenomyotic lesions. However, according to Dr. Liang, the normal uterine tissue survives because dormant collateral vessels will open up and feed the healthy tissue when the uterus senses a lack of oxygen after the UAE procedure. He explains that this phenomenon only occurs in healthy uterine tissue, not in adenomyotic lesions; therefore, the adenomyotic lesions will shrink and die, leaving only scar tissue. The particles used in

UAE will not block these collateral blood vessels because the particles are too big and are not able to enter them.

According to Dr. Liang, UAE is an effective treatment option for women with adenomyosis who do not wish to undergo a hysterectomy. However, not enough information is available at this time regarding Dr. Liang's UAE procedure and future pregnancy. If the patient wishes to become pregnant in the future, this procedure may ot be the best option. For more information on this procedure and how it affects future pregnancy, please contact Dr. Liang's office (see Appendix III).

Uterine Polyps

"She made broken look beautiful and strong look invincible. She walked with the universe on her shoulders and made it look like a pair of wings."

-Ariana Dancu

Uterine polyps are growths that form from the inner lining of the uterus (endometrium). They are attached to the uterine wall either by a thin stalk or a broad base. Also referred to as endometrial polyps, their size can range from a few millimeters to a few centimeters. They are most common in women in the fourth and fifth decade of life, and they are rare in women under 20 years of age. According to the Cleveland Clinic (2020), "estrogen...appears to be linked to the growth of uterine polyps."

Polyps are quite common and one of the most common causes of abnormal uterine bleeding, also known as AUB. They are typically benign but can rarely become malignant. Depending on their placement inside the uterine cavity, they may play a role in infertility. Polyps are known to occur in women with adenomyosis. According to Kanthi et al. (2016), risk factors for the development of polyps include hypertension, obesity, and tamoxifen use.

Symptoms of uterine polyps include infertility, irregular or heavy periods, bleeding between periods, bleeding after menopause, and bleeding after intercourse. Khanti et al. (2016) noted that the patients in their study also complained of "lower abdominal pain, backache, vaginal discharge, pruritis vulva, and hirsutism." Hirsutism refers to excessive hair growth in women.

Polyps can be easily diagnosed through TVS. A sonohysterogram (a procedure in which saline is infused into the uterine cavity followed by ultrasound) can aid in diagnosis. Other options include an endometrial biopsy or curettage.

In a study by Kanthi et al. (2016), women aged 40 to 49 years were the ones mostly affected by polyps. In addition, 45.6% of the women presented with AUB. Interestingly, 52% of the women had other reproductive abnormalities including fibroids, adenomyosis, ovarian cysts, infertility, polycystic ovarian syndrome, and dysfunctional uterine bleeding (DUB).

The gold standard of treatment is hysteroscopy; however, it is common for polyps to return after treatment.

Xenoestrogens

"Over four hundred pesticides are currently licensed for use on America's foods, and every year over 2.5 billion pounds are dumped on crop lands, forests, lawns, and fields."

-Burton Goldberg

Xenoestrogens are manufactured chemicals that have estrogen-like activity in the human body. They are considered dangerous because they can cause endocrine disruption (altering the function of hormones) which can lead to a whole host of reproductive health problems. Some scientists and doctors believe that xenoestrogens are harmless to humans and animals because we are routinely exposed to low levels of these chemicals without any adverse effects. However, it has been shown that the effects of xenoestrogens are additive, and if we are continually exposed to low levels of many different xenoestrogens, it could lead to health problems. According to a study by Bulayeva and Watson (2004), low levels of these chemicals may be more toxic than previously thought. The researchers state, "these very low effective doses for xenoestrogens demonstrate that many environmental contamination levels previously thought to be subtoxic may very well exert significant signal- and endocrine-disruptive effects, discernable only when the appropriate mechanism is assayed."

Some of the most dangerous xenoestrogens are herbicides and pesticides. Elizabeth Lipski (2000) states in her book, *Digestive Wellness,* "The average person consumes one pound of these chemicals each year. These pesticides have neurotoxic effects and can cause damage to our nervous systems."

An interesting study was done in Maine called The Body Burden Study. According to Marcelle Pick in her book, *Is it Me or My Hormones*, the researchers "decided to conduct a study...in which they had themselves tested for heavy metals. To their astonishment, they discovered that every single one of them had abnormally elevated levels of these toxic compounds.

The following is a list of some of the most dangerous and recognized xenoestrogens. Some of these chemicals have been banned, but many are still being used today. Also, some of the banned chemicals are still present in the environment since they do not break down easily. It is recommended that women who suffer from adenomyosis and endometriosis educate themselves on these chemicals and although impossible to avoid completely, try to do their best to decrease exposure where possible.

4-methylbenzylidine camphor (4-MBC) – This chemical is used in sunscreen. In addition to being an endocrine disruptor, it may also play a role in hypothyroidism. Margaret Schlumpf headed a study in Zurich, Switzerland at the Institute of Pharmacology and Toxicology in 2008. She and her colleagues found that 4-MBC applied to rat skin doubled the rate of growth of uterine tissue before puberty. Its use is approved in Europe and Canada, but it is banned in the U.S. and Japan.

Alkyl phenols (nonylphenols) – These chemicals have been shown to have clear estrogen activity. They are found in adhesives, carbonless copy paper, detergents, fire retardant materials, fragrances, fuels, lubricants, oil field chemicals, and tires. The use of alkyl phenols in Europe is restricted. For more information, see Bisphenol A (BPA).

Atrazine – This chemical is an herbicide that is used on corn, sugarcane, and other crops to control weed growth. It has also been used on golf courses and lawns. In 2004, atrazine was the second most widely used herbicide in the U.S., and it is the most commonly detected herbicide in drinking water. It is a persistent environmental pollutant which means it can persist in the environment for years. Studies have shown it to be an endocrine disruptor; however, the Environmental Protection Agency (EPA) reports levels are low enough that it probably won't cause reproductive problems. This statement has been criticized, however, and its safety is currently controversial. Tyrone B. Hayes from the University of California at Berkeley (2003) looked at the effect of atrazine on frogs. With increasing exposure to this chemical, some of the frogs began to show both male and female sex organs.

Benzophenone – a well-known UV filter, this substance is used in the printing industry and in sunscreens. It is also used in perfumes and soaps to prevent UV light from damaging their colors and scents. A study by Kunisue et al. (2012) examined some benzophenone derivatives and their role in endometriosis. The group looked at five benzophenone derivatives in the urine of 625 women in Utah and California. Six hundred of these women had undergone a laparoscopy, laparotomy, or pelvic MRI for possible endometriosis between 2007 and 2009. Adjusted odds ratios were calculated for benzophenone derivative urinary concentrations and the odds of an endometriosis diagnosis. They were able to find an association between endometriosis and one specific benzophenone derivative, namely 2,4-OH-BP (2,4-dihydroxybenzophenone). Several studies have already pointed to the potent xenoestrogen activity of 2,4-OH-BP. One such study was performed by Morohoshi et al. in 2005. This group was able to demonstrate estrogenic activity of several benzophenone derivatives. According to the authors, "Eleven compounds, most of which were benzophenone derivatives and parabens, showed binding affinity to ER [estrogen receptor] by ER-ELISA without s9 mix." According to Kunisue et al. (2012), "In vitro studies using recombinant yeast cells that express human ERα [estrogen receptor alpha] with the B-galactosidase reporter gene demonstrated an approximate 5-fold higher estrogenic activity of 2,4-OH-BP than bisphenol A (BPA), which is a well-known EDC [endocrine disrupting chemical]."

Bisphenol A (BPA) – This chemical is a substance that is used to make epoxy and plastic resins. Because of its moldability, durability, and heat resistance, it has been found to be quite useful in things like CDs, DVDs, food and beverage cans, sports equipment, and water bottles. About 20% of BPAs are used to line the interior of plastic containers and water bottles.

The major exposure route in humans is through the diet, and it is known to be an endocrine disruptor. It easily accumulates in fatty tissue.

In 2013, the Food and Drug Administration reported that BPA is safe at low levels; however, as of 2014, debates persist on its safety. BPA has been banned for use in baby bottles in Canada and Europe. In addition to being an endocrine disruptor, BPAs may play a role in cancer, diabetes, heart disease, neurological problems, and obesity.

Sadly, we also need to be wary of products labeled "BPA-free". The following is an excerpt from a blog that I wrote several years ago regarding BPS, a chemical touted at the time for being a safe alternative to BPS:

> In the last ten years or so, the safety of BPA has come into question. Studies have shown that it is an endocrine disruptor. In particular, it has been shown to interfere with estrogen receptors. Because of this concern, years of discussion ensued in governmental agencies worldwide leading to a ban of BPA use in the production of baby bottles and other products in children under the age of three. Today, some of these products are listed as "BPA-free".
>
> However, a study from the University of Texas pointed out that many "BPA-free" products now contain BPS, or bisphenol S. BPS is now being used as a substitute for BPA. Shockingly, this study shows that BPS is also an endocrine disruptor as it also interferes with estrogen receptors, so according to this study, "BPA-free" is NOT safe. As I continued to do my research, I found an article from Walsh (2011) that stated "Almost all commercially

available plastic products we sampled, independent of the type of resin, product, or retail source, leached chemicals having reliably detectable [endocrine activity], including those advertised as BPA-free. In some cases, BPA-free products released chemicals having more [endocrine activity] that BPA-containing products."

Butylated hydroxyanisole (BHA) – This chemical is a petroleum by-product that acts as an antioxidant and is used as a food preservative. Specifically, it prevents fats from becoming rancid. It can be found in cosmetics, medications, and rubber. BHA is known to be present in ice cream, shortening, candy, dry cereal, crackers, seasonings, instant potatoes, and animal food. Several studies have suggested that BHA is an endocrine disruptor. The National Institutes of Health report BHA is reasonably anticipated to be carcinogenic due to outcomes of some animal studies; however, in humans, the low intakes do not appear to show an increased risk. This chemical may irritate the liver, and some people may be allergic to it.

Dichlorobenzene – This endocrine disruptor is a pesticide, deodorant and disinfectant and is probably carcinogenic. Dichlorobenzene is not easily broken down and can build up in fatty tissues in the body. In addition, 1,3-dichlorobenzene has been found to have adverse effects on the thyroid and pituitary glands. Exposure comes from breathing the air where it is present. This chemical can be found in mothballs and in toilet deodorizer blocks.

Dichlorodiphenyltrichloroethane (DDT) – DDT is an insecticide that is classified as "moderately toxic." It builds up in fatty tissues and is considered a persistent environmental pollutant.

This chemical is a known endocrine disruptor and has been linked to menstrual disorders and other reproductive problems. Studies have also linked it to several types of cancer. A study done by toxicologist Michael Fry at the University of California Davis (1995) found female cells in the reproductive tracts of male gulls after they were injected with DDT, DDE, and methoxychlor (all xenoestrogens).

Its use was banned in 1972.

Dieldrin – This chemical is an insecticide that was used from the 1950s to the 1970s as an alternative to DDT. Specifically, farmers used this chemical to kill pests on crops, and it was used in homes to kill termites. It does not easily break down, and it is toxic to both humans and animals. Dieldrin can be found today in the soil. Plants can absorb it, and it can be found in the fat of animals. In addition to dieldrin being a probable carcinogen, it has been linked to reproductive disorders, breast cancer, and Parkinson's disease. It is banned from use in most parts of the world. Those at highest risk are people who live in old homes where this chemical was used to treat termites in the past or those who live near a hazardous waste site.

Diethylstilbestrol (DES) - This is a synthetic estrogen that was used in the U.S. between 1940 and 1975 to prevent miscarriage. Herbst et al. (1990) was able to connect clear cell vaginal adenocarcinoma with the use of DES. Harris & Waring (2012) and Troisi et al. (2013) showed that reproductive disorders such as uterine abnormalities and hormone-dependent cancers occurred in both male and female children of mothers who took DES. Alwis et al. (2011) showed that exposure to DES caused endometrial dysplasia and hyperplasia in female rats and hamsters.

DES was banned from use in 1971.

Dioxins – Dioxins are persistent environmental pollutants. They were produced in substantial amounts in the 20th century during industrial processes. Although the U.S. has reduced the production of these dangerous pollutants nearly 90 percent in the last 30 years or so, they are still produced through burning processes including backyard burning, incineration, wood/coal burning, cigarette smoking, or the eruption of volcanos. These chemicals consist of 210 chlorinated hydrocarbon compounds that are divided into 75 PCDDs (polychlorinated dibenzo-dioxins) and 135 PCDFs (polychlorinated dibenzo-furans). The most toxic of these is TCDD (2,3,7,8-tetrachlorodibenzodioxin). This is the dioxin involved in the industrial accident that occurred in Seveso, Italy, and it has been linked to the herbicide Agent Orange which was used during the Vietnam War to strip leaves from trees. Humans are most commonly exposed to dioxins via food, and most of the exposure comes from dairy, meat, fish, and shellfish.

These dangerous chemicals are resistant to degradation. The half-life of dioxins is 11.5 years, so dioxins can persist and build up in fatty tissue such as the breast. In fact, in Belgium, TCDD levels in breast milk are known to be remarkably high, and interestingly, this country has one of the highest levels of endometriosis in the world.

Rier et al. (2001) showed that chronic exposure to TCDD and other dioxin-like PCBs is associated with an increased risk of endometriosis in rhesus monkeys. The degree of endometriosis was dependent on the level of contamination. Yang et al. (2000) showed that TCDD exposure helped endometrial implants to grow in cynomolgus monkeys. Mayani et al. (1997) determined TCDD levels in the serum of infertile women who underwent diagnostic laparoscopy. They found a significantly higher level of this dioxin in women with endometriosis compared to those who didn't have the disease. Su et al. (2012) showed that dioxins can cause uterine structural abnormalities in 8 years old girls.

Nayer et al. (2006) showed that TCDD treatment in mice induced endometriosis and resulted in decreased expression of progesterone receptors and transforming growth factor beta 2 (TGFβ2). Of note, both TGFβ2 and progesterone receptors are also known to be reduced in adenomyosis. Although this study strongly suggests that TCDD induces endometriosis, according to Anger and Foster (2008), a mouse model is not ideal because mice do not go through a luteal phase of the menstrual cycle, do not develop endometriosis spontaneously, and must be immune deficient to perform this kind of study.

Simsa et al. (2010) conducted a study where they took plasma samples from 96 women with endometriosis and 106 control patients. They assessed the levels of dioxin-like compounds present in the plasma samples and concluded that "...women exposed to higher plasma concentrations of [dioxin-like compounds] were at higher risk of having endometriosis than women exposed to lower concentrations of [dioxin-like compounds] within normal environmental conditions." Porpora et al. (2006) showed that women with endometriosis had higher levels of dioxin-like and non-dioxin-like PCB residues compared to controls.

However, a few studies have not made this connection between endometriosis and dioxins. Eskenazi et al. (2002) followed a group of 601 women who were exposed to TCDD in Seveso, Italy and found that there was a non-significant risk of endometriosis in this study group. However, a limitation of this study was that endometriosis was not confirmed by laparoscopy, and women who had symptoms were included but may have been suffering from a condition other than endometriosis. Pauwels et al. (2001) found a statistically insignificant association between blood dioxin levels and endometriosis.

In the above cases, endometriosis was not classified into peritoneal or deep nodule endometriosis. Therefore, Heilier et al. (2005) performed a study in which they divided the women into separate groups (peritoneal, deep nodule, etc.) and used fertile women as their control group. They also took age, parity, breast-feeding, and body mass index (BMI) into account when analyzing their results. BMI is important to consider since it is known that TCDD can build up in fatty tissue. It is known that

TCDD body burden can be reduced in those who have had children and/or are breast-feeding. They found that PCDDs and PCDFs were associated with significant disease risk. Dioxin-like PCBs were associated with an increased risk of disease in patients only with deep endometriotic (adenomyotic) nodules.

Progesterone resistance comes into play here. Bruner-Tran et al. (2010) has linked TCDD exposure to a progesterone-resistant phenotype in endometriosis. Bruner-Tran et al. (2010) state, "Although TCDD is known to have both estrogenic and antiestrogen activity, our research suggested that disruption of progesterone action may be a more critical factor in determining the early establishment of peritoneal sites of endometrial growth." They summarize by stating, "In general, we find that exposure of the human endometrium to TCDD acts to promote a similar progesterone-resistant endometrial phenotype that we and others have observed in tissues acquired from women with endometriosis."

Endosulfan – Endosulfan is an insecticide that treats infestations of whiteflies, aphids, and leafhoppers. It is one of the most toxic pesticides known to man, and its use is being discontinued on a global scale. Currently, in the U.S., endosulfan cannot be used in residential homes. The levels of this chemical are regularly monitored in the U.S. by state and federal agencies. In addition to being neurotoxic to both humans and animals, it is an endocrine disruptor. According to The Agency for Toxic Substances and Disease Registry (ATSDR, 2018), "Two studies of environmental exposure of humans suggested that endosulfan may be associated with alterations in the levels of thyroid hormones and some sex hormones in the blood." However, they also state that in these studies, participants were also exposed to other pesticides, so it cannot be determined if endosulfan was entirely responsible for these hormonal effects. Most exposure comes by way of diet.

Ethinyl estradiol – Ethinyl estradiol is the estrogen component of birth control pills. It is released into the environment as a xenoestrogen through the urine and feces of women who take these pills. This leads to a conundrum. Endometriosis and adenomyosis patients take birth control pills as a treatment for the disorders, but the use of them increases xenoestrogens in the environment which may make the occurrence of these disorders more common. This emphasizes the urgency for research to come up with treatment options that prevent an increase in xenoestrogen levels in the environment.

Hepatachlor – This chemical is an insecticide that smells like camphor. It was used in homes, building, and on food crops. It has not been used for these purposes since 1988, but it can stick to soil and persist in the environment for decades. It is still cleared for use to kill fire ants in underground power transformers, but it is not clear if it is still being used for that purpose. Hepatachlor can be found in breast milk, dairy products, drinking water, fish, shellfish, poultry, and meat. In addition to being a possible carcinogen, hepatachlor may have a negative impact on fertility and the nervous system. Animal studies have shown that high exposure can cause liver damage and a decrease in fertility.

Gamma-hexachlorocyclohexane (Lindane) – Lindane is an organochlorine pesticide (OCP) that has been used on humans as a treatment for lice and scabies. β-hexachlorocyclohexane (β-HCHis a by-product of lindane and has been shown to be a possible endocrine disruptor and carcinogen. Interestingly, a study done in 2013 showed an increased risk of endometriosis in women who were found to have high blood serum levels of β-HCH (Upson et al., 2013). The women with the highest levels of β-HCH in their blood serum were thirty to seventy percent more likely to have endometriosis than the women with the lowest levels of this chemical in their serum. In addition, in the same study, the researchers found a slight link between another OCP (Mirex) and endometriosis. Mirex was used in the 1960s and

1970s as an insecticide against fire ants. Lindane was banned from use in 2009 except for use as a last resort in the treatment of lice and scabies. However, because Lindane and Mirex are stable and persist in the environment, these two chemicals are still of concern today. Upson et al. (2013) concluded "extensive past use of environmentally persistent OCPs in the United States or present use in other countries may affect the health of reproductive-age women."

Metalloestrogens – These substances have an affinity for estrogen receptors and are therefore possible endocrine disruptors. They also potentially play a role in breast cancer. The following are known metalloestrogens: (add more specifics on each one)

- Aluminum – Correia et al. (2010) studied the effects of this metalloestrogen in Nile tilapia fish. Control fish were exposed to acidic water, and the concentration of plasma 17α hydroxyprogesterone increased. The opposite effect was seen in female fish exposed to aluminum. In addition, the cortisol levels in these female fish exposed to aluminum was decreased.
- Antimony – Plastic beverage bottles in the United States contain a plastic called polyethylene terephthalate (PET). Antimony is used in the polycondensation of PET. According to Sax et al. (2010), both antimony and phthalates can leach from PET bottles, and the higher the temperature, the more leaching that occurs. In addition, Choe et al. (2003) has shown that antimony has high estrogenic activity.
- Arsenite – Davey et al. (2007) reports that arsenic is a potent endocrine disruptor that alters gene function of glucocorticoids, mineralocorticoids, progesterone and androgen steroid receptors. Arsenic also disrupts ER in

both cell culture and in vivo. The group states, " Arsenic (As) contamination of drinking water is considered a serious worldwide environmental health threat..."

- Barium – Choe et al. (2003) states that barium is possibly estrogenic. Kwon et al. (2016) subjected zebrafish to barium chloride and found that it could, "modulate gene transcription and hormone production of the [hypothalamus-pituitary-gonadal] axis in a sex-dependent way which could cause adverse effects on reproduction..."
- Cadmium – This metalloestrogen is used in batteries, plastics, and metallic pigments. It is known to accumulate in the liver and kidneys. Cadmium is also a known endocrine disruptor with potent estrogen and androgen-like activities. It affects steroid synthesis in reproductive organs and can cause an increase in fetal death and placental necrosis. Takiguchi et al. (2006) report that high levels of cadmium have been reported in women with fibroids (in whole blood).
- Cobalt – High levels of cobalt have been seen in women with fibroids (Johnstone et al., 2014).
- Copper – Cao et al. (2019) showed that exposure of zebrafish to increasing levels of copper altered "the steroid hormone levels and the expressions of endocrine related genes in the [hypothalamus-pituitary-adrenal axis] of zebrafish." In addition, Martin et al. (2003) showed that copper accumulates in uterine and mammary tissue and modulates sensitivity of these tissues to estrogen and antiestrogens. It has been shown that in women, an increase in estrogen levels during pregnancy is linked to increased levels of circulating copper.
- Lead – This metalloestrogen is used in paint, oil, and toys. In addition to being an endocrine

disruptor, lead can cause abnormalities in brain development. Johnstone et al. (2014) states that increased levels are seen in whole blood in women with fibroids. In addition, Martin et al. (2003) states that lead has been linked to an increase in menstrual cycle disturbances, infertility, miscarriage, preeclampsia, and other reproductive issues.

- Mercury – This metalloestrogen is used in industrial processes. Burning charcoal can emit mercury, and human exposure can come from eating fish. In human and animals, mercury affects the function of the pituitary, thyroid, adrenals, and pancreas. Mercury can alter the levels of FSH, LH, estrogen, progesterone and androgens. According to Rice et al. (2014), "There is good evidence linking mercury with menstrual disorders including abnormal bleeding, short, long, irregular cycles, and painful periods."
- Nickel - see allergy section for more detailed information.
- Selenite – A study by Stoica et al. (2000) has shown that selenite interacts with the hormone binding domain of the ERα receptor.
- Tin – Martin et al. (2003) showed tin has a significant effect on the ERα expression/activity. It has been shown to induce the growth of Mcf-7 breast cancer cells. The authors state, "The ability of metals to bind with high affinity and activate ERα suggests that at environmentally relevant doses, these compounds may pose a risk for endocrine-related diseases."
- Vanadate – Martin et al. (2003) showed vanadate has a significant effect of ERα expression/activity. Specifically, it activates ERα receptor through its hormone binding domain. In addition, vanadate has been shown to induce the growth of Mcf-7 breast cancer cells.

Methoxychlor – Methoxychlor is an insecticide that was used as an alternative to DDT. It was used to kill insects and other pests including mosquitos, flies, and cockroaches. This chemical was used on agricultural crops and animal feed. It is known to stick to soil; however, it does not appear to build up in the food chain because it is broken down easily in fish and animals. Methoxychlor is not usually found in food or water, and exposure is more likely to occur in those living near a hazardous waste site.

Methoxychlor is a known endocrine disruptor. According to the ATSD (2018), "Studies in animals show that exposure to methoxychlor adversely affects the ovaries, uterus, and mating cycles in females..." They also note that fertility is also decreased with exposure to this chemical.

Methoxychlor is banned from use.

Parabens – These chemicals are preservatives used in cosmetics, moisturizers, shampoos, shaving cream, and toothpaste. Parabens are used in cosmetics because they do not cause irritation or allergy. They are also used in baked goods, artificial sweeteners, and diet foods. They have weak estrogen activity and have been linked to early menarche in young girls. Engeli et al. (2017) tested multiple parabens to see if they inhibited 17-β-HSD-1 (estrogen-activating) and 17-β-HSD-2 (estrogen-inactivating). All tested parabens inhibited 17-β-HSD-2. Some of them size-dependently decreased 17-β-HSD. Of note is that parabens are rapidly metabolized into the inactive p-hydroxybenzoic acid. This must be kept in mind when evaluating the effects of parabens in vivo. More studies are needed.

Pentachlorophenol – This chemical is a pesticide and a disinfectant. It is used in wood preservation, paper mills, and masonry. Pentachlorophenol can be found in leather and rope, and the EPA reports it is probably carcinogenic. It is rapidly metabolized, so buildup in the environment is probably not a big issue. Today this chemical is primarily used on utility poles and railroad ties, and it is treated as regulated hazardous waste in the United States. Studies have shown that pentachlorophenol is an endocrine disruptor and interferes with thyroid function.

Phthalates – Phthalates are chemicals that are added to plastics to increase flexibility (plasticizer). Three types of phthalates have been shown to have estrogenic effects: di(2-ethylhexyl phthalate (DEHP), benzyl-butyl phthalate (BBP), and dibutyl phthalate (DBP). DEHP is the most common phthalate and is used specifically in medical products such as tubing, blood bags, dialysis equipment and disposable gloves. It can also leach from hospital IV bags. DEHP is broken down in the body into mono-(2-ethylhexyl) phthalate (MEHP).

Phthalates can be found in adhesives, building supplies, butter, caulk, children's toys, detergents, eye shadow, food containers, floor tiles, hair spray, meats, medication, milk, nail polish, nutritional supplements, packaging materials, paints, printing ink, shower curtains, and upholstery.

Phthalates have been shown to be endocrine disruptors in studies in rats. Kim et al. (2011) showed that increased levels of the phthalates DEHP and MEHP were higher in the plasma of women with endometriosis when compared to disease-free controls. Huang et al (2010) showed that women with endometriosis had significantly higher urinary levels of the phthalate mono-n-butyl phthalate as compared to controls. In addition, Buck Louis et al. (2013) showed that in women with endometriosis, levels of six phthalate metabolites were twice as high as controls. Hart et al. (2014) showed that exposure to mono (carboxy-isoctyl) phthalate changed uterine volume in women with endometriosis. Reddy et al. (2006) looked at phthalate levels in infertile women with severe endometriosis and used fertile women without endometriosis as controls. The women with severe endometriosis had higher levels of four phthalates, including DEHP, in their plasma. However, this same observation was not seen with MEHP.

However, there have been studies that refute the above findings. The study by Reddy et al. mentioned above has a drawback. DEHP is rapidly metabolized in the body. Therefore, the MEHP level would be expected to be much higher than was observed while the DEHP level should have been lower if there was a link to endometriosis. Therefore, the results of that study should be considered cautiously. In fact, Anger and Foster (2008) suggest that metabolites of DEHP should be studied in women with endometriosis instead of DEHP levels to get more accurate results. Additionally, Upson et al. (2013) found that MEHP reduced the risk of developing adenomyosis. Itoh et al. (2009) confirmed this in a study of infertile women; however, there were very few participants in this study.

Anger and Foster (2008) report that DEHP decreases circulating estradiol in rats while MEHP decreases aromatase mRNA and protein expression. Since both estradiol and aromatase are known to be elevated in adenomyosis and endometriosis, one would conclude that phthalates are not the cause this disorder based on this study. However, it is not a good idea to completely rule out phthalates at this point as they may promote the growth of endometriosis via another pathway. Further superior quality clinical studies are needed.

Europe and the U.S. have restricted the use of phthalates in children's toys.

Phenosulfonphthalein (Phenol red) – This chemical is a red dye that is used in laboratory media as a PH indicator. Phenol red is also found in some home swimming pool test kits. It is a known weak endocrine disruptor.

Polybrominated biphenyls (PBBs) - Polybrominated biphenyls (PBBs) are used a flame retardant. They were used in electrical products, plastic foam, rugs, textiles, and upholstery.

Manufacturing of PBBs stopped in 1976 in the U.S.; however, these chemicals do not break down easily in the environment and tend to accumulate. Exposure usually comes from eating contaminated food or living near hazardous waste sites.

PBBs are possible menstruation disruptors. In one study, young girls who were exposed to elevated levels of PBBs were shown to start menstruating at an earlier age.

Polychlorinated biphenyls (PCBs) – PCBs are endocrine disruptors that affect the thyroid hormone and cause estrogenic and anti-androgenic activity. PCBs imitate and inhibit estradiol in the body which may lead to all kinds of menstrual and reproductive disorders and cancers. They are carcinogenic and have been banned from use since 1979.

Polychlorinated biphenyls were first manufactured in the 1920s and were used in paint, adhesives, rubber, and resin industries. They were also used in carbonless copy paper, caulk, cements, hydraulic fluids, lubricating oils, paints, and pesticides. PCBs were used extensively which resulted in heavy contamination of the environment. These chemicals do not readily decompose and are considered persistent environment pollutants. They are lipophilic which means they accumulate in fatty tissue. According to Anger and Foster (2008), 90 percent of human exposure is through diet. PCBs are particularly high in fish, meat, milk, and eggs.

Overall, the clearest connection between endometriosis development and PCBs was through those that had dioxin-like activity (see dioxins). In addition, Dr. Elena De Felip et al. published a study in 2006 in which 80 women with endometriosis were evaluated for levels 11 different PCB congeners. They showed that the levels of these congeners were 1.6 times higher in women with endometriosis than in the control group. They also showed that PCB 138, 153, and 180 were particularly high in these women. Those three congeners are known to have estrogenic activity.

However, Buck Louis (2005) showed that 4 PCB congeners that are anti-estrogenic were 3 times higher in women with endometriosis in her study group. She states, "We don't fully understand the role of estrogenic and antiestrogenic PCBs." According to Potera (2006), conflicting data may be a "result of complex interactions of many PCBs as well as other chemicals...."

More research is needed to definitively determine the effects of PCBs on the endocrine system.

Propyl gallate – This synthetic chemical is an antioxidant added to fats and vegetable oils as a preservative. Specifically, it protects against rancidity by preventing oxidation. It can be found in non-food items such as adhesives, bath products, cosmetics, hair care products, lubricants, sunscreen, and toothpaste. Propyl gallate can also be found in foods such as microwavable popcorn, cereal, chewing gum, and soups. Several studies have shown propyl gallate to be a possible endocrine disruptor.

Sodium lauryl sulfate (SLS) – This chemical is a surfactant that causes cleaning items to foam. SLS is quite often contaminated with the dangerous chemical 1,4-dioxane. The FDA recommends limits on 1,4-dioxane content in cosmetics but has not established a specific limit. SLS can be found in bubble baths, cleaning products, some food products, laundry detergents, pesticides, shampoo, shaving cream, and toothpaste. It can be irritating to the eyes, skin, and respiratory tract, and prolonged exposure may cause dermatitis. In addition, SLS is possibly carcinogenic.

Triclosan – This chemical is an antibacterial and antifungal agent that is often used in hospitals, and it is especially useful to use when dealing with patients with MRSA (methicillin-resistant staphylococcus aureus) infections. Its safety is under review in both the U.S. and Canada. Studies have shown that excessive exposure to triclosan may cause a reduction in thyroid hormone levels.

Triclosan can be found in deodorants, detergents, hospital scrubs, mouthwash, shampoo, soaps, cosmetics, and toothpaste. This chemical can also be found in non-food items such as clothing, furniture, and toys.

The MIREC Study of Maternal-Infant Research on Environmental Chemicals, which included about 2000 women in the first trimester of pregnancy who were exposed to phthalates at the time of conception, showed that exposure to elevated levels of triclosan decreased fertility.

Conclusion

"I went downstairs to our pathologist's office in Boston. I said, 'Show me the textbook that you actually find as the best textbook for pathology of the female reproductive tract.' There's an entire textbook edited by George Mettler at Brigham. Out of 400 pages in this entire book on the female reproductive tract, there is one full page on adenomyosis."

-Keith Isaacson, MD

Education, proper diagnosis, better treatment options, and more research are necessary to treat both endometriosis and adenomyosis patients effectively.

Education:

It is vitally important to educate not only the doctors but also family, friends, co-workers, and others about both endometriosis and adenomyosis. The Endometriosis Foundation of America has a program (The ENPOWR Project) to educate teenagers in school about these disorders. Not only girls, but also boys, need to understand these conditions so that future patients will have the support of their significant others. Of note, a patient in a study done by Moradi et al. (2014) stated, "In school, we've never heard of endometriosis...even when I did biology and science." The women in this study suggested the following to improve knowledge and understanding of endometriosis:

- Increase knowledge of general practitioners about the disease.
- Educating students at school.
- Increase support groups/networks
- Society needs to achieve a better understanding of the disease and acceptance without criticism or stigmatization

Endometriosis diagnosis and treatment:

The most effective way to learn the proper treatment of both adenomyosis and endometriosis patients is to listen to the top experts in the field.

Dr. Camran Nezhat (2021), one of the world's most well-known endometriosis surgeons, states, "Endometriosis is not just a reproductive tract disease, but one which can potentially cause severe chronic symptoms throughout the entire body, including incapacitating pain, severe chronic fatigue, infertility, immune and endocrinologic dysfunction, and damage to multiple organs and tissues, including the bowel, bladder, ureters, diaphragm, muscles, musculoskeletal structures, nerves, ligaments, lungs, and liver."

Dr. Tamer Seckin (2020) explains how he questions women who may have endometriosis and/or adenomyosis. He asks them about the frequency of their periods, the amount of bleeding, how regular their periods are, if there is any ovulatory pain (mittelschmerz). He asks about any bladder symptoms, if they have any pain with sex or any pain the day after sex. He asks about leg pain, hip pain, and even chest pain that may occur during their period. One of the most important questions that he asks is about bowel function, specifically diarrhea alternating with constipation, painful bowel movements, bloating, vomiting, cramps. It is also very telling to him when the bowel symptoms worsen around the time of the woman's period. When these symptoms flare up around a woman's period, it is highly suggestive of endometriosis.

If conservative management fails, surgery should be considered. According to Dr. Tamer Seckin (2020), the surgery should be excision surgery and not electrocautery or ablation. He also explains that care should be taken to remove all endometriotic lesion. He states, "If you remove 99% lesion and leave one, it is like a mini electrical circuit. And they, with even one single stimulus, will press the button, pain centers that had developed for 10 years. It will evoke the same potential of pain in the patient."

Dr. Ken Sinervo (2016) points out that the sooner a patient is diagnosed with endometriosis, the better the prognosis. Early diagnosis will improve quality of life and physical symptoms, and it will improve the patient's chances of obtaining and maintaining a healthy pregnancy. He states, "...what matters most is the skill of the provider, their understanding of the disease and fertility-sparing principles, and of course – the patient's needs above all else."

Adenomyosis diagnosis and treatment:

Dr. Ketih Isaacson (2019) explains why it is so hard to diagnose adenomyosis. "We have no standardized histologic definition. We have no standardized radiologic definition. The diagnosis is most often made without a tissue diagnosis...We have no standard classification of the disease, so it is hard for us to communicate with each other as to what stage one, two three, or four diseases. It is all descriptive."

Dr. Ketih Isaacson (2019, Endometriosis Foundation of America) explains that physicians are taught that adenomyosis occurs in women in their 40s and that women at highest risk are those who have had multiple children. "Why is that?" he asks. "Those are risk factors not for adenomyosis I'd say. Those are risk factors for the patient who is going to have a hysterectomy...I think we've missed the disease early on in their adult life." He also makes an excellent point as we move forward in our research of adenomyosis. As you will see in a following section, many enzymes, proteins, etc. have all been shown to be abnormally high or low in adenomyosis. Although these are extremely important findings, Dr. Isaacson suggests that we need to look at these results through systems biology. We must remember that all these enzymes, proteins, etc. are all interrelated, and when we just focus on one substance, thinking that one thing is the cause of adenomyosis, we are not going to make much progress. This disease is probably the result of many different abnormalities, and we need to research how these all work together to develop this disease state. He states, "we have to have systems like this if we're gonna make any headway on understanding the disease."

Additional hormone testing:

As shown through my own cortisol testing and through clinical studies of cortisol levels in women with endometriosis, aberrant cortisol levels may be observed in these women. It is known that aromatase is elevated in these disorders, and high cortisol levels are known to increase aromatase levels. One study mentioned in this book found that serum cortisol levels (total cortisol) was found to be significantly higher in women with endometriosis as compared to controls.

Aluminum is a metalloestrogen and a xenoestrogen. One study showed that cortisol levels in Nile tilapia fish exposed to aluminum were lower than in the same type of fish that were not exposed to aluminum.

Finally, multiple clinical studies have shown low cortisol levels (hypocortisolism) in saliva samples (free cortisol) in women with endometriosis. Because of these results, it is imperative that gynecologists include adrenal hormone blood tests when evaluating women with suspected adenomyosis and endometriosis.

Final conclusion:

As the reader can see through my story, my case was mismanaged. The most important clue was excruciatingly painful bowel movements that occurred during menstruation. Other clues included infertility, a high MPV value which could have indicated platelet aggregation, painful intercourse and pain in the back of my vagina during a pelvic exam which could have indicated rectovaginal endometriosis, and failure to test appropriate hormone levels (progesterone was never tested during those entire 17 years). All of these clues should have alerted my doctors to the possibility of endometriosis and/or adenomyosis.

Laparoscopic ablation of endometrial lesions is no longer advised, and when I had this surgery, it was ineffective. The endometrial ablation failed in my case; however, at the time, I did not know I had adenomyosis, so it technically was not contraindicated. We now know that an endometrial ablation is not recommended in adenomyosis, but surprisingly, many patients are being told that an ablation should be done in adenomyosis cases. Women on the Adenomyosis Fighters Support Group Facebook page report that their doctors are still pushing endometrial ablation to this day. This is not acceptable and is simply a result of lack of education.

Finally, as Dr. Eisen Liang states in his book, *Could It be Adenomyosis? The (Bad) Cousin of Endometriosis (2021)*, "It took generations to achieve recognition of endometriosis as a REAL problem. Adenomyosis is just as common, and arguably more debilitating. Now is the time to speak about adeno."

Appendix I

Summary of my pharmaceutical and surgical treatments

Anesthetic:

Bupivicaine
General anesthesia – 12 times

Birth control pills:

Two unknown brands
Ortho Novum 777®
Orthocyclen®
Yasmin®
Lo Estrin®

Blood thinners:

Plavix
Heparin

Pain relievers:

Motrin®/ibuprofen
Tylenol®
Imitrex®
Gabapentin
Vicodin® (hydrocodone)
Percocet®
Ponstel® (mefenamic acid)

Muscle relaxers:

Levsin®
Bentyl®
Robaxin® (methocarbamol)
Flexeril®
Valium® (diazepam)

Fertility drugs:

Clomid®

Antidepressants:

Prozac® (Sarafem®)
Zoloft®
Cymbalta® (duloxetine)
Effexor® (venlafaxine)
Paxil® (paroxetine)

Acid reflux medication:

Prilosec®

Antihistamines:

Claritin®
Zyrtec®
Astelin® (azelastine) nasal spray
Nasocort® nasal spray
Flonase® nasal spray
Benadryl®

Antibiotics:

Biaxin® (clarithromycin)
Levaquin® (levofloxacin)
Zithromax® (azithromycin)
Cipro® (ciprofloxacin)
Avelox® (moxifloxacin)
Ancef® (cefazolin)
Clindamycin
Vancomycin
Doxycycline

Statin:

Crestor®

Steroids:

Prednisone
Depo-medrol® (methylprednisolone)
Decadron® (dexamethasone)
Multiple steroid shots in knee, back, and hip

Vitamins:

Multivitamin
Folate
Calcium
Prescription vitamin D – 50,000 IU once per week

Other natural treatments:

Metamucil
Prune juice
Fiber
Flaxseed
Fish oil

Other:

Anusol HC® (rectal hydrocortisone cream)
Nitroglycerine cream (used for anal fissure)
Allergy shots
Dulcolax®
Fleet® enema
Saline nasal rinses
Bengay®
Singulair® (montelukast)
Preparation H®
Monistat®
Zantac®
Mylanta®
Magnesium citrate

Surgeries:

1 D&C (dilation and curettage)
Laparoscopy
Hysteroscopy
Endometrial ablation
Hysterectomy
3 spinal fusions
Cholecystectomy
Brain aneurysm coil and stent
Knee arthroscopy

Diagnostic tests:

Hysterosonogram
Multiple transvaginal ultrasounds
Multiple Pap smears and pelvic exams
Multiple blood draws for hormone levels, CBC, metabolic panel,
        autoimmune tests, etc.
Repeated treatment by physical therapists
Multiple X-rays
Multiple MRIs
Several CAT scans

Appendix II

Summary of abnormalities seen in adenomyosis as per clinical studies

I decided to add this section to demonstrate how clinical studies have shown that there are actual abnormalities that have been documented in adenomyosis. The following list includes substances such as enzymes and proteins, along with abnormalities in certain pathways, that have been shown in studies to be either upregulated, downregulated, overly expressed or under expressed. The purpose of this list is to show that this disorder is not psychological, as some physicians have told their patients. There are actual documented abnormalities that have been seen in this disorder.

Upregulated/overly expressed:

Cox-2 – cyclooxygenase 2
Erβ (estrogen receptor beta)
Erα (estrogen receptor alpha)
Aromatase
Oxytocin
NFkB p65
NFkB p50
NFkB p52
DNMT1
DNMT3B
HDAC1
HDAC3
TGF-β (tissue growth factor beta)
Myostatin
Follistatin
Activin A
FAK (focal adhesion kinase)
Annexin A2
RhoA/Rock-1 signaling
IL-1B (interleukin 1B)

CRH
UCN (urocortin)
IL-10 (interleukin 10)
NGF-B (nerve growth factor B)
SYN (synaptophysin)
MAP2 mRNA
Bcl-2
EGF (epidermal growth factor)

Downregulated/under expressed:

PRB (progesterone receptor B)
IkB-2 immunoreactivity
CAV1 (caveolin)
GAD 65-expressing neurons
GRIM-19 (retinoid-interferon-induced mortality 19)
HOX10A
NR4A
FOXO1A
Integrin B3
OPN (osteopontin)

In addition to the above abnormalities, local hyperestrogenism
has been noted along with the presence of highly aggregated
platelets. Progesterone receptor B has also been shown to be
hypermethylated which renders it silent and results in
progesterone resistance. See Platelet Aggregation and Estrogen
Dominance for more detailed information.

Appendix III

Recommended Facilities for Endometriosis and Adenomyosis Treatment

Center for Endometriosis Care
> Dr. Ken Sinervo, Medical Director
> 6105 Peachtree Dunwoody Road
> Building B, Suite 230
> Atlanta, GA 30328
> Phone: (770)913-0001
> www.centerforendo.com
> **Colorectal resection expert

Center for Innovative GYN Care
> Multiple locations:
>
> 3206 Tower Oaks Blvd.
> Suite 200
> Rockville, MD 20852
>
> 1860 Town Center Dr.
> Suite 255
> Reston, VA 20190
>
> 352 7th Ave.
> Suite 1202
> New York, NY 10001
>
> 325 Claremont Ave.
> Suite 100
> Montclair, NJ 07042
>
> Phone: 1-888-418-4038
> www.innovativegyn.com

Endometriosis Foundation of America

Founders: Dr. Tamer Seckin and Padma Lakshmi
872 5th Ave.
New York, NY 10065
Phone: (212)988-4160
www.endofound.org
**Colorectal resection expert

Camran Nezhat Institute

1775 Woodside Rd.
Suite 202
Woodside, CA 94061
Phone: (650)327-8778
www.nezhat.org
**Colorectal resection expert

Sydney Fibroid Clinic

UAE experts for adenomyosis
Dr. Eisen Liang, founder
4 locations:

St. Leonards:
Suite 305
St. Leonards Square
480 Pacific Hwy.
St. Leonards NSW 2065

Wahroonga:
Suite 407
San Clinic, Sydney Adventist Hospital
185 Fox Valley Road
Wahroonga NSW 2076

Bella Vista:
Suite 107
Norwest Private Hospital Medical Centre

9 Norbrik Drive
Bella Vista NSW 2153

Westmead:
Suite 5
Westmead Private Hospital
Corner Mons and Darcy Road
Westmead NSW 2145

www.sydneyfibroidclinic.com.au
(02)9480 8729

Appendix IV

Recommended books

Could it be Adenomyosis? The (Bad) Cousin of Endometriosis: An Unsuspected Cause of Heavy Painful Periods by Dr. Eisen Liang with Dr. Bevin Brown

The Doctor Will See You Now: Recognizing and Treating Endometriosis by Dr. Tamer Seckin and Padma Lakshmi

What You Must Know About Women's Hormones: Your Guide to Natural Hormone Treatments for PMS, Menopause, Osteoporosis, PCOS, and More by Dr. Pamela W. Smith

Is It Me or My Hormones? The Good, the Bad and the Ugly About PMS, Perimenopause, and All the Crazy Things That Occur with Hormone Imbalance by Marcelle Pick, MSN, OB/Gyn NP

Acronyms

4-MBC - 4-methylbenzylidine camphor

5-HIAA – 5-hydroxyindoleacetic acid

17β-HSD type 2 – 17-beta hydroxysteroid dehydrogenase type 2

α-SMA – alpha smooth muscle actin

ALA – alpha lipoic acid

ALP – alkaline phosphatase

APC – antigen-presenting cell

ATSDR – Agency for Toxic Substances and Disease Registry

AUB – abnormal uterine bleeding

BBP – benzyl-butyl phthalate

BCL-2 – B-cell lymphoma 2

BCP – birth control pill

β-HCH - β-hexachlorocyclohexane

BMI – body mass index

BMP-2 – bone morphogenic protein 2

BPA – Bisphenol A

BHA -butylated hydroxyanisole

CA 125 – cancer antigen 125

CAV1 – caveolin

CBC – complete blood count

CIGC – Center for Innovative GYN Care

CMP – comprehensive metabolic panel

CO2 – carbon dioxide

COX-1 – cyclooxygenase 1

COX-2 – cyclooxygenase 2

CRH – corticotropin-releasing hormone

CRP – c-reactive protein

CT - CAT scan

D&C – dilation and curettage

DBP – dibutyl phthalate

DDT – dichlorodiphenyltrichloroethane

DEHP – di(2-ethylhexyl) phthalate

DES - diethylstilbestrol

DHEA – dehydroepiandrosterone

DIE – deep infiltrating endometriosis

DNG – dienogest

DNMT – DNA methyltranserase

DUB – dysfunctional uterine bleeding

DVT - deep vein thrombosis

E1 – estrone

E2 – estradiol

E3 – estriol

ECM – extracellular matrix

EDC – endocrine disrupting chemical

EFA – essential fatty acid

EGF – epidermal growth factor

EMG - electromyography

EMI – endometrial/myometrial interface, AKA junctional zone

EMT – epithelial to mesenchymal transition

EPA – Environmental Protection Agency

ERα – estrogen receptor alpha

ERBβ – estrogen receptor beta

ERCP – endoscopic retrograde cholangiopancreatography

FAK – focal adhesion kinase

FDA – Food and Drug Administration

FMT – fibroblast to myeloblast transdifferentiation

FOXO1A – forkhead box 1A

FSH – follicle stimulating hormone

GAD-65 – glutamic acid decarboxylase 65 kilodalton isoform

GERD – gastroesophageal reflux disease

GHBT – glucose hydrogen breath test

GnRHa – gonadotropin-releasing hormone agonists

GRIM-19 – retinoid-interferon induced mortality 19

HBT – hydrogen breath test

HDAC – histone deacetylase

HOXA10 – homeobox A10

IBS – irritable bowel syndrome

IC – interstitial cystitis
ICSI – intracytoplasmic sperm injection
IFN - interferon
IgE – immunoglobulin E
IgG – immunoglobulin G
IgM – immunoglobulin M
****IkB-2** - confirm this!!
IL-1B – interleukin 1B
IL-4 – interleukin 4
IL-5 – interleukin 5
IL-6 – interleukin 6
IL- 10 – interleukin 10
IL-12 – interleukin 12
IL-13 –interleukin 13
IUD – intrauterine device
IV - intravenous
IVF – in vitro fertilization
JZ – junctional zone
LH – luteinizing hormone
LOX - lipoxygenase
MEHP – mono(2-ethylhexyl) phthalate
MIREC – Maternal-infant Research on Environmental Chemicals
MPV – mean platelet volume
MRI – magnetic resonance imaging
mRNA – messenger ribonucleic acid
MRSA – methicillin-resistant staphylococcus aureus
MVD – microvessel density
NFkB – nuclear factor kappa B
NGF-β - nerve growth factor beta
NIH – National Institutes of Health
NK – natural killer
NR4A – orphan nuclear receptor 4A
NSAID – non-steroidal anti-inflammatory drug
OCD – obsessive-compulsive disorder
OCP – oral contraceptive pill or organochlorine pesticide

OPN – osteopontin
OTC – over the counter
PBB – polybrominated biphenyl
PCB – polychlorinated biphenyl
PCDD – polychlorinated dibenzo-dioxins
PCDFs - polychlorinated dibenzo-furans
PCNA – proliferating cell nuclear antigen
PCOS – polycystic ovarian syndrome
PCR – polymerase chain reaction
PDW – platelet distribution width
PG – prostaglandin
pJNK – c-Jun N-terminal kinase
PMDD – premenstrual dysphoric disorder
PMS – premenstrual syndrome
POP – persistent organic pollutant
PRα – progesterone receptor α
PRβ - progesterone receptor β
RVE – rectovaginal endometriosis
SDG – secoisolariciresinol diglucoside
SIBO – small intestine bacterial overgrowth
SLS - Sodium lauryl sulfate
SMM – smooth muscle metaplasia
SSRI – selective serotonin reuptake inhibitor
SYN - synaptophisin
TAC – total antioxidant capacity
TCDD - 2,3,7,8-tetrachlorodibenzodioxin
TGF-β1 - transforming growth factor beta 1
Th1 – T-helper cell 1
Th2 – T-helper cell 2
TIAR – tissue injury and repair
TNF-α - tumor necrosis factor alpha
TSH – thyroid-stimulating hormone
TVUS – transvaginal ultrasound
TXA2 – thromboxane A2
UAE – uterine artery embolization
UAL – uterine artery ligation

UCN - urocortin
US – ultrasound
VEGF – vascular endothelial growth factor
VMA – vanillyandelic acid
WHI – Women's Health Initiative

Definition of terms

5-HIAA – a substance formed from the breakdown of serotonin in the liver. Low levels are seen in depression, OCD, and other disorders.

17β hydroxysteroid dehydrogenase type 2 (17β HSD type 2) - An enzyme that inactivates androgens and estrogens. It can also activate 20α-hydroxyprogesterone which results in the production of the more potent progesterone.

Adenomyoma – abnormal mass of endometrial tissue found within the myometrium. An adenomyoma is usually benign and is associated with adenomyosis.

Adhesion – abnormal union of two separate tissues due to inflammation.

Androgen - a type of sex hormone. It is made by both sexes, but more is made in the male. DHEA and testosterone are androgens. In women, androgens can be converted into estradiol.

Antigen – a foreign substance that is presented to an antigen-presenting cell (APC) for destruction and removal from the body.

Antioxidant – a substance that inhibits oxidation reactions.

Apoptosis – programmed cell death.

Aromatase – an enzyme that converts androgens to estrogens

B-cell lymphoma 2 (Bcl-2) - a protein encoded by the B-cell lymphoma gene that regulates cell death (apoptosis).

β-HCH – this organochloride is a by-product of Lindane (an insecticide) and is considered a persistent organic pollutant (POP). It has been linked to Parkinson's disease and Alzheimer's disease.

Benign – not cancerous.

Biopsy – removal of a small piece of tissue from the body. It is then analyzed under a microscope to determine if an abnormality is present.

Birth control pill - a contraceptive pill that usually contains both a progestin and an estrogen. It is taken daily for three weeks, and then a sugar pill is taken for one week during which a withdrawal bleed occurs (menstruation).

Cancer antigen 125 (CA125) - marker that detects the initial stages of ovarian cancer; however, this marker is elevated in other conditions such as endometriosis and adenomyosis, so it is now considered a non-specific test that is not useful in the diagnosis of endometriosis and adenomyosis.

Cervix – cylindrical shaped tissue that separates the body of the uterus from the vagina. The cervix contains uterine tissue (explain).

Chemokine - a type of cytokine that is active during inflammation and stimulate the action of white blood cells.

C-Jun N-terminal kinase (pJNK) - kinases that respond to stresses I the body. For purposes of this book, pJNKs respond to the activity of cytokines.

Comprehensive metabolic panel (CMP) - a blood test that assesses the chemical balance and metabolism in the body. It includes 14 tests including glucose, sodium, potassium, chloride, calcium, protein, carbon dioxide, 5 liver function tests (albumin, ALP, AST, ALT, and bilirubin, and 2 kidney tests (BUN and creatinine).

COX-1 – also called cyclooxygenase 1, this enzyme speeds up the production of prostaglandins in certain areas of the body including the stomach. This promotes inflammation.

COX-2 - also called cyclooxygenase 2, this enzyme speeds up the production of prostaglandins at the sites of inflammation. It is responsible for inflammation and pain. Unlike COX-1, it is not active in the stomach.

Cystic – related to or containing cysts.

Cytochrome P450 – hemoproteins that are involved in the metabolism of toxins in the body. Most of these hemoproteins are found in the liver.

Cytokine - small proteins important in cell signaling. Interleukins, chemokines, interferon, and tumor necrosis factor are all types of cytokines. They are very important in the proper functioning of the immune system.

DHEA – precursor to testosterone and estrogen.

Dienogest (DNG) - a semi-synthetic progestin. It has been used to treat endometriosis under the name Visanne.

Dilation and curettage (D&C) - a surgical procedure in which the cervix is dilated, and the physician scrapes away any abnormal tissue from inside the uterus (curettage). This procedure is commonly used to treat heavy or prolonged menstrual bleeding.

Dyschezia – Difficult and/or painful defecation.

Dysmenorrhea – painful menstrual bleeding.

Dysuria - Difficult and/or painful urination

E-cadherin - also known as epithelial cadherin, it is a type of CAM (cell adhesion molecule) that is involved in cell-cell adhesion. E-cadherin is also a tumor suppressor protein.

Ectopic – occurring in an abnormal place; out of proper position.

Eicosanoid - signaling molecules derived from polyunsaturated fatty acids, usually arachidonic acid. Prostaglandins, thromboxanes, leukotrienes, lipoxins are all examples of eicosanoids. These substances are active in many different bodily processes such as regulating inflammation, allergic responses, and fever regulation. They are also active in the reproductive, vascular, renal, and GI systems.

Endocrine disrupting chemicals (EDCs) – chemicals that cause hormonal imbalance by interfering with the proper functioning of the endocrine system. Xenoestrogens are endocrine disruptors.

Endometrial ablation – a surgical procedure that destroys the inner layer of the uterus, also known as the endometrium.

Endometrial biopsy – a procedure in which a thin tube is inserted into the uterus via the cervix, and a small piece of the endometrium is removed. This sample is sent to the laboratory for examination.

Endometrium – the innermost lining of the uterus that responds to hormonal stimulation.

Eosinophil - a type of white blood cell that is usually involved in allergic reactions.

Eotaxin - type of chemokine that attracts eosinophils.

Epidermal growth factor (EGF) - a protein that stimulates cell growth.

Essential fatty acid (EFA) - fats that cannot be synthesized by the human body and must be included in the diet.

Estradiol (E2) – the most potent form of estrogen produced by the human body. It is the predominant form of estrogen during the reproductive years. The level of estradiol drops after menopause.

Estriol (E3) - a type of estrogen that is produced by the placenta and is abundant during pregnancy.

Estrogen – sex hormone responsible for the development and maintenance of female characteristics and reproduction. Plays a key role in the menstrual cycle. There are 3 forms of estrogen – estrone (E1), estradiol (E2), and estriol (E3).

ERα - estrogen receptor alpha is a nuclear receptor that is activated by estrogen. It is found in many tissues throughout the body, and it is one of two major estrogen receptors. According to Paterni et al. (2014), this receptor is more abundant in mammary glands, uterus, ovary, bone, liver, and fat in women. It appears to be most active in mammary glands, uterus, in the skeleton, and in regulating metabolism.

ERβ - estrogen receptor beta is a nuclear receptor that is activated by estrogen. It is found in many tissues throughout the body, and it is one of two major estrogen receptors in humans. According to Paterni et al. (2014), this receptor is most abundant in the bladder, ovary, colon, and fatty tissue, and it is highly active in the immune system and the central nervous system. It also counteracts the action of ERα in the breast and uterus.

Estrone (E1) - the least abundant type of estrogen. It is less potent than estradiol and is the major form of estrogen found in menopausal women. Estrone can be converted into estradiol in the body.

Fallopian tube – the tube connecting the ovary to the uterus. The egg travels down this tube after being released from the ovarian follicle at ovulation.

Fibrinogenesis - Process of production of fibrin (protein formed as a result of blood clotting).

Fibrocystic breast disease – non-cancerous cysts in the breast. The cysts can be solid (fibrosis) or fluid-filled, and their growth is stimulated by estrogen.

Fibroid – a benign tumor of the uterine smooth muscle (myometrium). Also referred to as a leiomyoma, it can cause heavy periods, infertility, and anemia.

Follicle stimulating hormone (FSH) – a hormone produced in the anterior pituitary gland that is responsible for the maturation of ovarian follicles.

Follistatin - a glycoprotein that inhibits the activity of activins. It is known to inhibit the action of TGF-β and FSH.

Glucose hydrogen breath test - also known as HBT, this test measures the amount of hydrogen produced after drinking a sugar solution. The patient typically fasts for 8 to 12 hours before the test. This test can detect the presence of small intestinal bacterial overgrowth (SIBO).

Gonadotropin – a hormone that stimulates the gonads. FSH and LH are examples of gonadotropins.

Gonadotropin-releasing hormone (GnRH) - this hormone is made in the hypothalamus. It stimulates the pituitary gland to make follicle-stimulating hormone and luteinizing hormone, and these two hormones stimulate the ovaries to make estrogen and progesterone.

Hirsutism – excessive male pattern hair growth in women.

Helminth – another term for a parasitic worm.

HOX genes – also known as homeobox genes, these genes determine the structure of an organism.

Hyperprolactinemia – higher than normal levels of prolactin in a woman's body. Can cause oligomenorrhea, amenorrhea, and infertility.

Hypertrophic – excessive growth of an organ or tissue.

Hysteroscopy – the examination of the inside of the uterus and the cervix using a small lighted instrument called a hysteroscope.

Interferon - a type of cytokine produced by the body in response to viruses. This cytokine interferes with viral replication.

Interleukin - a type of glycoprotein produced by white blood cells that regulates immune responses.

Interleukin-6 (IL-6) - a protein produced by T-lymphocytes in response to infection and injury. It causes B-cells to mature which results in an increase in the production of antibodies. It is known to cause chronic inflammation when its production is not well-controlled within the body. It is also known to be a pyrogen (causes fever).

Interstitial cystitis (IC) - a condition that causes increased pressure and pain within the bladder.

Intrauterine device (IUD) - a small plastic device that is placed into a woman's uterus to prevent pregnancy. This small t-shaped device prevents the sperm from fertilizing the egg.

In vitro fertilization (IVF) – a medical procedure where eggs and sperm are combined in the laboratory, allowed to grow into embryos, and then either inserted into the woman's uterus or frozen.

Irritable bowel syndrome (IBS) – disorder of the colon that can cause abdominal pain, cramping, bloating, constipation, and/or diarrhea. IBS is a diagnosis of exclusion which means that the physician must rule out all other known causes of these symptoms before this diagnosis can be assigned. IBS is a functional disorder of the colon due to abnormal peristalsis (wave-like contractions), and it is not life-threatening. Adenomyosis and endometriosis are known to commonly be misdiagnosed as IBS.

Junctional zone (JZ) – the area in between the endometrium and the myometrium in the uterine wall. Also known as EMI, or the endometrial-myometrial interface.

Laparoscopic supracervical hysterectomy – a type of hysterectomy in which only the uterus is removed. The cervix stays intact.

Laparoscopy – a procedure that used a long, thin, rod-like structure, called a laparoscope, to view the inside of the abdomen. Usually, three or four incisions are made. The incision at the belly button is where the laparoscope is inserted. The laparoscope has a lens and light to aid viewing the abdominal cavity. Small instruments are inserted in the other incisions which aid in performing the actual surgery.

Leiomyoma – another term for a uterine fibroid.

Luteinizing hormone (LH) – a hormone produced in the anterior pituitary gland. A surge in LH occurs in the last half of the menstrual cycle and is responsible for ovulation and the development of the corpus luteum.

Macrophage – a type of large white blood cell that is involved in the destruction of foreign invaders such as bacteria and viruses. It is a major player in the functioning of the immune system.

Magnetic resonance imaging (MRI) - a machine that uses a powerful magnet in addition to radio waves to create noticeably clear pictures (more detailed than other imaging devices) of organs, tissues, bones, etc. Inside the body.

Menarche – the first menstrual cycle.

Menorrhagia – abnormally heavy menstrual bleeding.

Meta-analysis - an analysis that uses statistics to combine findings from two or more studies.

Müllerian ducts - embryonic ducts that develop into fallopian tubes, uterus cervix, and vagina.

Myometrium – The outer muscular layer of the uterus.

Myostatin – a type of growth factor that regulates the size of muscles.

Non-steroidal inflammatory drug (NSAID) - a medication used to treat pain and inflammation. Depending on specific NSAID, they block either COX-1 or COX-2 or both.

Oligomenorrhea – infrequent or noticeably light menstrual periods.

Oxytocin – a hormone that helps to regulate childbirth and breast-feeding. It is produced in the hypothalamus and stored in the posterior pituitary gland.

Peristalsis – involuntary rhythmic contractions that move contents through a tubular organ such as the intestines.

Pesticide – a chemical that kills any kind of pest. Herbicides and insecticides are two types of pesticides.

Pituitary gland – a pea-sized gland located at the base of the brain. It controls the functioning of endocrine glands and is involved in the production of several different hormones in the body. Also referred to as the "master gland."

Polycystic ovarian syndrome (PCOS) - an ovarian disorder in which many small cysts develop on the ovaries. This is due to a hormonal imbalance caused by excessive levels of androgens. Symptoms include excess body hair, weight gain, infertility, and irregular periods.

Premenstrual dysphoric disorder (PMDD) – a severe form of premenstrual syndrome (PMS).

Premenstrual syndrome (PMS) – a group of symptoms that some women experience just prior to menstruation. Symptoms include moodiness, bloating, irritability, anxiety, depression, fatigue, insomnia, and headache.

Progesterone – female sex hormone that plays a significant role in the menstrual cycle.

Prolactin – a hormone synthesized by the pituitary gland (confirm) that stimulates the production of breast milk.

Prostaglandin – a type of lipid that controls the contraction and relaxation of smooth muscle, modulates inflammation, and regulates blood flow. It is made from arachidonic acid, a type of omega-6 fatty acid. Prostaglandins are a type of eicosanoid.

Smads – proteins important in regulating cell growth. They are signal transducers for TGFβ1.

Small intestinal bacterial overgrowth (SIBO) - Also called blind loop syndrome, this condition occurs when excess bacteria, including bacteria not normally seen, is present in the small intestine.

Smooth muscle metaplasia (SMM) - transformation of non-smooth muscle cells into smooth muscle cells.

Sonohysterogram – a special type of ultrasound which uses saline infused into the uterus to obtain a better picture of the inside of the uterus than regular ultrasound. This test is also called saline infusion sonography (SIS).

Speculum – an instrument that looks like the "beak of a duck" and is used to spread open the walls of the vagina during a pelvic examination by a gynecologist.

Testosterone – a male sex hormone. It is also present in tiny amounts in females.

Thyroid – an endocrine gland that makes and stores hormones.

Thyroid stimulating hormone (TSH) - a hormone produced in the pituitary gland that stimulates the release of thyroid hormone.

Transvaginal ultrasound (TVS) - a type of ultrasound used to view the uterus, fallopian tubes, and ovaries. The probe is inserted into the vagina to view these organs.

Tubal insufflation – a procedure where a gas, usually carbon dioxide is injected transvaginally into the uterus to see if the fallopian tubes are open.

Tumor necrosis factor - a pro-inflammatory cytokine that regulates immune cells, causes fever, is active in apoptosis (programmed cell death), and is involved in many other functions.

Ultrasound - also called a sonogram, an ultrasound is a procedure that uses sound waves to visualize organs and tissues inside the body.

Uterine hyperperistalsis – a condition where uterine contractions are more frequent than those seen in a normal uterus.

Uterine implantation – the adherence of a fertilized egg to the wall of the uterus.

Uterine polyp – mass that originates from the endometrium. It can be flat up against the uterine wall or it may be pedunculated (on a stalk). Polyps can grow up to several centimeters and may be associated with heavy menstrual bleeding. Also referred to as an endometrial polyp.

Vanillyandelic acid (VMA) - breakdown product of epinephrine and norepinephrine.

References

Agency for Toxic Substances & Disease Registry (2018). Public Health Statement for Endosulfan. Retrieved from www.atsdr.cdc.gov/phs/phs.asp?id=607&tid=113

Agency for Toxic Substances & Disease Registry (2018). Public Health Statement for Methoxychlor. Retrieved from www.atsdr.dcd.gov/phs/phs.asp?id=776&tid=151

Albee, R. B. (2016). Adenomyosis: Is it Really Endometriosis? Center for Endometriosis Care. Retrieved from www.centerforendo.com/adenomyosis-is-it-really-endometriosis

Alwis, I.D., Maroni, D.M., Hendry, I.R., Roy, S.K., May, J.V., Leavitt, W.W., & Hendry, W.J. (2011). Neonatal diethylstilbestrol exposure disrupts female reproductive tract structure/function via both direct and indirect mechanisms in the hamster. *Reprod Toxicol, 32(4),* 472-83. doi: 10.1016/j.reprotox.2011.09.006

Anger, D.L. & Foster, W.G. (2008). The link between environmental toxicant exposure and endometriosis. *Frontiers in Bioscience, 13,* 1578-1593. doi: 10.2741/2782

Attia, G.R., Zeitoun, K., Edwards, D., Johns, A., Carr, B.R., & Bulun, S.E. (2000). Progesterone receptor isoform A but not B is expressed in endometriosis. *J Clin Endocrinol Metab, 85,* 2897-902. doi: 10.1210/jcem.85.8.6739

Badaway, A.M., Elnashar, A.M., & Mosbah, A.A. (2012). Aromatase inhibitors or gonadotropin-releasing hormone agonists for the management of uterine adenomyosis: A randomized controlled trial. *Acta Obstericia Gynecologica Scandivavica, 91,* 489-495. doi: 10.1111/j.1600-0412.2012.01350.

Bazot, M., Cortez, A., Darai, E., Rouger, J., Chopier, J., Antoine, J.M., & Uzan, S. (2001). Ultrasonography compared with magnetic resonance imaging for the diagnosis of adenomyosis: Correlation with histopathology. *Human Reproduction, 16(11),* 2427-33. Retrieved from https:// ncbi.nlm.nih.gov/pubmed/1167953

Beelen, P., Reinders, I., Scheepers, W., Herman, M., Geomini, P., Van Kuijk, S., & Bongers, M. (2019). Prognostic factors for the failure of endometrial ablation: A systematic review and meta-analysis. *American Journal of Obstetrics & Gynecology, 134(6),* 1269-1281. doi: 10.1097/AOG.0000000000003556

Benagiano, G.P., Brosens, I.A., Carrara, S., & Filippi, V. (2010). Adenomyosis. *The Global Library of Women's Medicine*, ISSN: 1756-2228. doi: 10.3843/GLOWM.10460

Bodur, S., Dundar, O., Pektas, M.K., Babayigit, M.A., Ozden, O., & Kucukodaci, Z. (2015). The clinical significance of classical and new emerging determinants of adenomyosis. *Int J Clin Exp Med, 8(5),* 7958-7964. Retrieved from https:// ncbi.nlm.nih.gov/pmc/articles/PMC 4509299/

Borghini, R., Porpora, M.G., Casale, R., Marino, M., Palmieri, E., Greco, N., Donato, G., & Picarelli, A. (2020). Irritable bowel syndrome-like disorders in endometriosis: Prevalence of nickel sensitivity and effects of a low-nickel diet. An open-label pilot study. *Nutrients, 12(2),*341. doi: 10.3390/nu12020341

Bromley, B., Shipp, T.D., & Benacerraf, B. (2000). Adenomyosis: Sonographic findings and diagnostic accuracy. *Journal of Ultrasound in Medicine,* 19, 529-534. Retrieved from https://www.jultrasoundmed. org/content/19/8/529.full.pdf

Bruner-Tran, K.L., Ding, T. & Osteen, K.G. (2010). Dioxin and endometrial progesterone resistance. *Semin Reprod Med, 28(1),* 59-68. doi: 10.1055/s-0029-1242995

Buck Louis, G.M., Peterson, C.M., Chen, Z., Croughan, M., Sundaram, R., Stanford, J., Varner, M., Kennedy, A., Guidice, L., Fujimoto, V.Y., Sun, L., Wang., L., Guo, Y. & Kannan, K. (2013). Bisphenol A and phthalates and endometriosis, the ENDO study. *Fertility and Sterility, 100(1),* 162-169.e2. doi: 10.1016/j.fertnstert.2013.03.026

Bulayeva, N. & Watson, C. (2004). Xenoestrogen-induced ERK-1 and ERK-2 activation via multiple membrane-initiated signaling pathways. *Environmental Health Perspectives, 112(15),* 1481-87. Retrieved from https://www.bvsde/paho.org/bvsacd/ehp/v112-15/p1481.pdf

Bulleti, C., Coccia, M.E., Battistoni, S., & Borini, A. (2010). Endometriosis and infertility. *J Assist Reprod Genet, 27(8)*, 441-447. doi: 10.1007/s10815-010-9436-1

Campo, S., Campo, V., & Benagiano, G. (2012). Infertility and adenomyosis. *Obstetrics and Gynecology International, Volume 2012*, article ID 786132. doi: 10.1155/2012/786132

Cao, J., Wang, G., Wang, T., Chen, J., Wenjing, G., Wu, P., He, X., & Xie, L. (2019). Copper caused reproductive endocrine disruption in zebrafish (Danio rerio). *Aquat Toxicol, 211*, 124-136. doi: 10.1016/j.aquatox.2019.04.003

Caserta, D., Mallozzi, M., Pulcinelli, F.M., Mossa, B., & Moscarini, M. (2015). Endometriosis allergic or autoimmune disease: Pathogenetic aspects – a case control study. *Clinical and Experimental Obstetrics and Gynecology, 43(3)*, 354-7. doi: 10.12891/ceog2122.2016

Center for Endometriosis Care (2021). The Endo-Belly Bloat – A Symptom of Endometriosis? Retrieved from https://centerforendo.com/endobelly

Center for Endometriosis Care (2022). Endometriosis: A Complex Disease. Retrieved from https:// centerforendo.com/endometriosis-understanding-a-complex-disease

Center for Endometriosis Care (2022). Excision of Endometriosis. Retrieved from https://centerforendo.com/lapex-laparoscopic-excision-of-endometriosis

Center for Innovative GYN Care (2021). Is Endometriosis Painful? Understanding the Types of Endo Pain. Retrieved from https://innovativegyn.com/blog/is-endometriosis-painful-understanding-the-types-of-endo-pain/

Center for Innovative Gyn Care (2022). What are Uterine Fibroids? Retrieved from https://innovativegyn.com/conditions/fibroids/

Chamani, S. ,Liberale, L., Mobasheri, L., Montecucco, F., Al-Rasadi, K., Jamialahmadi, T., & Sahebkar, A. (2021). The role of statins in the differentiation and function of bone cells. *European Journal of Clinical Investigation, 51(7)*, E13534. doi: 10.1111/eci.13534

Chaudhari, R.K., Mahla, A.S., Singh, A.K., Singh, S.K., Pawde, A.M., Gandham, R.K., Singh, G., Sarkar, M., Kumar, H. & Krishnaswamy, N. (2018). Effect of dietary n-3 polyunsaturated fatty acid fish oil on the endometrial prostaglandin production in the doe. *Prostaglandins and Other Lipid Mediators, 135,* 27-35. doi: 10.1016/j.prostaglandins.2018.02.001

Cho, S., Nam, A., Kim, H., Chay, D., Park, K., Cho, D.J., Park, Y. & Lee, B. (2008). Clinical effects of the levonorgestrel-releasing intrauterine device in patients with adenomyosis. *American Journal of Obstetrics and Gynecology, 198 (4),* 373.el-7. doi:10.1016/ajog.2007.10.798

Choe, S.Y., Kim, S.J., Hae-Gyoung, K., Lee, J.H., Choi, Lee, H., & Kim, Y. (2003). Evaluation of estrogenicity of major heavy metals. *Sci Total Environ, 312(1),* 15-21. doi: 10.1016/S0048-9697(03)00190-6

Ciavattini, A., Serri, M., Carpini, G.D., Morini, S., & Clemente, N. (2016). Ovarian endometriosis and vitamin D serum levels. *Gynecological Endocrinology, 33(2),* 164-167. doi: 10.1080/09513590.2016.1239254

Cirillo, D.J., Wallace, R.B., Rodabough, R.J., Greenland, P., LaCroix, A. Z., Limacher, M.C., & Larson, J.C. (2005). Effect of estrogen therapy on gallbladder disease. *Journal of the American Medical Association, 293(3),* 330-339. doi: 10.1001/jama.293.3.330

Cleveland Clinic (2021). Menstrual Migraines (Hormone Headaches). Retrieved from https:// my.clevelandclinic.org/health/diseases/8260-menstrual-migraines-hormone-headaches

Cleveland Clinic (2022). Uterine Polyps. Retrieved from https:// my.clevelandclinic.org/health/diseases/14683-uterine-polyps

Correia, T.G., Narcizo, A.M., Bianchini, A., & Moreira, R.G. (2010). Aluminum as an endocrine disruptor in female Nile tilapia (Oreochromis niloticus). *Comp Biochem Physiol C Toxicol Pharmacol, 151(4),* 461-6. doi: 10.1016/j.cbpc.2010.02.002

Danilyants, Natalya (2022). Groundbreaking Minimally Invasive GYN Surgery. Retrieved from https:// innovativegyn.com/techniques/dualportgyn/

Davey, J.C., Bodwell, J.E., Gosse, J.A., & Hamilton, J.W. (2007). Arsenic as an endocrine disruptor: Effects of arsenic on estrogen-receptor-mediated gene expression in vivo and in cell culture. *Toxicological Sciences, 98(1)*, 75-86. doi: 10.1093/toxsci/kfm013

DeSouza, N.M., Brosens, J.J., Schwieso, J.C., Paraschos, T., & Winston, R.M. (1995). The potential value of magnetic resonance imaging in infertility. *Clinical Radiology, 50(2),* 75-9. Retrieved from https://www.ncbi.nlm.nih.gov/pubmed/7867272

Dueholm, M., Lundorf, E., Hansen, E.S., Sorensen, J.S., Ledertoug, S., & Olesen, F. (2001). Magnetic resonance imaging and transvaginal ultrasonography for the diagnosis of adenomyosis. *Fertility and Sterility, 76,* 588-594. doi: 10.1016/S0015-0282(01)01962-8

El-Kader, A.I.A., Gonied, A.S., Mohamed, M.L., & Mohamed, S.L. (2019). Impact of endometriosis-related adhesions on quality of life among infertile women. *Int J Fertil Steril, 13(1),* 72-76. doi: 10.22074/jifs.2019.5572

Endometriosis Foundation of America (2015). An Interview with Dr. Tamer Seckin, Endo Expert. Retrieved from https:// endofound.org/an-interview-with-dr-tamer-seckin-endo-expert

Endometriosis Foundation of America (2022). Endometriosis Treatment and Support. Retrieved from endofound.org/endometriosis-treatment-support

Engeli, R.T., Rohrer, S.R., Vuorinen, A., Herdlinger, S., Kaserer, T., Leugger, S., Schuster, D., & Odermatt, A. (2017). Interference of paraben compounds with estrogen metabolism by inhibition of 17β-hydroxysteroid dehydrogenases. *Int J Mol Sci, 18(9).* doi: 10.3390/ijms/8092007

Eskenazi, B., Mocarelli, P., Warner, M., Samuels, S., Vercellini, P., Olive, D., Needham, L.L., Patterson, D.G., Brambila, P., Gavoni, N., Casalini, S., Panazza, S., Turner, W., & Gerthoux, P.M. (2002). Serum dioxin concentrations and endometriosis: A cohort study in Seveso, Italy. *Environmental Health Perspectives, 110(7),* 629-34. doi: 10.1289/ehp.02110629

Exacoustos, C., Brienza, L., DiGiovanni, A., Szaboles, B., Romanini, M.E., Supi, E., & Arduini, D. (2011). Adenomyosis: Three dimensional sonographic findings of the junctional zone and correlation with histology. *Ultrasound in Obstetrics and Gynecology, 37(4),* 471-9. doi: 10.1002/uog.8900

Fedele, L., Bianchi, S., Zanconato, G., Portuese, A., & Raffaelli, R. (2001). Use of a levonorgestrel-releasing intrauterine device in the treatment of rectovaginal endometriosis. *Fertility and Sterility, 75,* 485-8. doi: 10.1016/s0015-0282(00)01759-3

Fong, Y.F. & Singh, K. (1999). Medical treatment of a grossly enlarged adenomyotic uterus with the levonorgestrel-releasing intrauterine system. *Contraception, 60(3),* 173-175. doi: 10.1016/S0010-7824(99)00075-X

Food and Drug Administration (2012). FDA Drug Safety Communication: Updated Information About the Risk of Blood Clots in Women Taking Birth Control Pills Containing Drospirenone. Retrieved from https://fda.gov/drugs/drug-safety-communication-update-information-about-risk-blood-clots-women-taking-birth-control

Fry, M. (1995). Reproductive effects in birds exposed to pesticides and industrial chemicals. *Environmental Health Perspectives, 103 (Suppl 7),* 165-171. Retrieved from https://www.ncbi.nlm.nih.gov/PMC/articles/PMC1518881/pdf/envhper00367-0160.pdf

Garavaglia, E., Serafini, A., Inversetti, A., Ferrari, S., Tandoi, I., Corti, L., & Candiani, M. (2015). Adenomyosis and its impact on women fertility. *Iran Journal of Reproductive Medicine, 13(6),* 327-336. Retrieved from www.ncbi.nlm.nih.gov /pmc/articles/PMC4555051/

Ghoshal, U.C. & Srivastava, D. (2014). Irritable bowel syndrome and small intestinal bacterial overgrowth: Meaningful association or unnecessary hype. *World J Gastroenterol, 20(10),* 2482-91. doi: 10.3748/wjg.v20.i10.2482

Ghoshal, U.C., Nehra, A., Mathur, A., & Rai, S. (2020). A meta-analysis on small intestinal bacterial overgrowth in patients with different subtypes of irritable bowel syndrome. *J Gastroenterol Hepatol, 35(6),* 922-931. doi: 10.1111/jgh.14938

Griffiths, A.N., Koutsouridou, R.N., & Penketh, R.J. (2007). Predicting the presence of rectovaginal endometriosis from the clinical history: A retrospective observational study. *J Obstet Gynaecol, 27(5),* 493-5. doi: 10.1080/01443610701405721

Haeggstrom, A., Ostberg, B., Stjerna, P., Graf, P., & Hallen, H. (2000). Nasal mucosal swelling and reactivity during a menstrual cycle. *ORL Journal for Oto-Rhino-Laryngology and Its Related Specialties, 62(1),* 39-42. doi: 10.1159/000027713

Harada, T., Taniguchi, F., Amano, H., Kurosawa, Y., Idena, Y., Hayashi, K., & Harada, T. (2019). Adverse obstetrical outcomes for women with endometriosis and adenomyosis: A large cohort of the Japan environment and children's study. *PLoS One, 14(8)*: e0220256. doi: 10.1371/journal.pone.0220256

Harris, R.M. & Waring, R.H. (2012). Diethylstilboestrol – A long-term legacy. *Maturitus, 72(2),* 108-12. doi: 10.1016/j.maturitas.2012.03.002

Hart, R., Doherty, D.A., Frederiksen, H., Keelan, J.A., Hickey, M., Sloboda, D., Pennell, C.E., Newnham, J.P., Skakkebaek, N.E., & Main, K.M. (2014). The influence of antenatal exposure to phthalates on subsequent female reproductive development in adolescence: A pilot study. *Reproduction, 147(4),* 379-90. doi: 10.1530/REP/13-0331

Hayashi, A., Tanabe, A., Kawabe, S., Hayashi, M., Yugushi, H., Yamashita, Y., Okuda, K. & Ohmichi, M. (2012). Dienogest increases the progesterone receptor isoform B/A ratio in patients with ovarian endometriosis. *J Ovarian Res, 5,* 31. doi: 10.1186/1757-2215-5-31

Hayes, T., Haston, K., Tsui, M., Hoang, A., Haeffele, C., & Vonk, A. (2003). Atrazine-induced hermaphroditism at 0.1 ppb in American leopard frogs (Ranna pipiens): Laboratory and field evidence. *Environmental Health Perspectives, 111(4),* 568-575. Retrieved from https://www.ncbi.nlm.nih.gov/pubmed/PMC1241446

Heilier, J.F., Nackers, F., Verougstraete, V., Tonglet, R., Lison, D., & Donnez, J. (2005). Increased dioxin-like compounds in the serum of women with peritoneal endometriosis and deep endometriotic (adenomyotic) nodules. *Fertility and Sterility, 84(2),* 305-12. doi: 10.1016/j.fertnstert.2005.04.001

Herbst, A.L. & Anderson, D. (1990). Clear cell adenocarcinoma of the vagina and cervix secondary to intrauterine exposure to diethylstilbestrol. *Semin Surg Oncol, 6(6),* 343-6. doi: 10.1002/ssu.2980060609

Huang, P.C., Tsai, E.M., Li, W.F., Liao, P.C., Chung, M.C., Wang, Y.H., & Wang, S.L. (2010). Association between phthalate exposure and glutathione s-transferase M1 polymorphism in adenomyosis, leiomyoma and endometriosis. *Human Reproduction, 25(4),* 986-94. doi: 10.1093/humrep/deq015

Isaacson, K., MD. (2019). Adenomyosis Dilemma. Endometriosis Foundation of America. Retrieved from https://www.endofound.org/keith-isaacson-md-adenomyosis-dilemma

Itoh, H., Iwasaki, M., Hanaoka, T., Sasaki, H., Tanaka, T., & Tsugane, S. (2009). Urinary phthalate monoesters and endometriosis in infertile Japanese women. *Science of the Total Environment, 408(1),* 37-42. doi: 10.1016/j.scitotenv.2009.09.012

Johnstone, E., Buck Louis, G., Parsons, P.J., Steuerwald, A.J., Palmer, C.D., Chen, Z., Sun, L., Hammoud, A.D., Dorias, J., & Peterson, C.M. (2013). Increased urinary cobalt and whole blood concentrations of cadmium and lead in women with uterine leiomyomata: Findings from the ENDO study. *Reproductive Toxicology, 49,* 27-32. doi: 10.1016/j.reprotox.2014.06.007

Kanthi, J.M., Remadevi, C., Sumathy, S., Sharma, D., Sreedhar, S., & Jose, A. (2016). Clinical study of endometrial polyp and role of diagnostic hysteroscopy and blind avulsion of polyp. *Journal of Clinical Diagnostic Research, 10(6),* QC01-QC04. doi: 10.7860/JCDR/2016/18173.7983

Keselman, A. & Heller, N. (2015). Estrogen signaling modulates allergic inflammation and contributes to sex differences in asthma. *Frontiers in Immunology, 6,* 568. doi: 10.3389/fimmu.2015.00568

Kalluri, R. & Weinbery, R. (2009). The basics of epithelial-mesenchymal transition. *The Journal of Clinical Investigation, 119(6),* 1420-1428. doi: 10.1172/JCI39104

Kalogeromitros, D., Katsarou, A., Armenaka, M., Rigopoulos, D., Zapanati, M., & Straitgos, I. (1995). Influence of the menstrual cycle on skin-prick test reactions to histamine, morphine, and allergen.

Clinical and Experimental Allergy, 25(5), 461-466. doi: 10.1111/j.1365-2222.1995.tb01078.x

Kim, S.H., Cun, S., Jang, J.Y., Chae, H.D., Kim, C.H., & Kang, B.M. (2001). Increased plasma levels of phthalate esters in women with advanced-stage endometriosis: A prospective case-control study. *Fertility and Sterility, 95(1),* 357-9. doi: 10.1016/j.fertnstert.2010.07.1059

Kimura, F., Takahashi, K., Takebayashi, K., Fujiwara, M., Kita, N., Noda, Y. & Harada, N. (2007). Concomitant treatment of severe uterine adenomyosis in a premenopausal woman with an aromatase inhibitor and a gonadotropin-releasing hormone agonist. *Fertility and Sterility, 87(6),* 1468.e9-12. doi: 10.1016/j.fertnstert.2006.09.010

Kirmaz, D., Yuksel H., Mete, N., Bayrak, P., & Baytur, Y.B. (2004). Is the menstrual cycle affecting the skin prick test reactivity? *Asian Pacific Journal of Allergy and Immunology, 22(4),* 197-203. Retrieved from https://pubmed.ncbi.nlm.nih.gov/15783132/

Kruse, C., Seyer-Hansen, M., & Forman, A. (2012). Diagnosis and treatment of rectovaginal endometriosis: An overview. *Acta Obstetricia et Gynecologica Scandivavica,91(6),* 648-657. doi: 10.1111/j.1600-0412.2012.01367.x

Kuivasaari, P., Hippelainen, M., Anttila, M. & Heinonen, S. (2005). Effect of endometriosis on IVF/ICSI outcome: Stage III/IV endometriosis worsens cumulative pregnancy and live-born rates. *Human Reproduction, 20(1),* 3130-3135. doi: 10.1093/humrep/dei176

Kunisue, T., Chen, Z., Buck-Louis, G., Dundaram, R., Hediger, M., Sun, L., & Kannan, K. (2012). Urinary concentrations of benzophenone-type UV filters in U.S. women and their association with endometriosis. *Environmental Science and Technology, 46(8),* 4624-4632. doi: 10.1021/es204415a

Kunz, G., Herbertz, M., Beil, D., Huppert, P., & Leyendecker, G. (2007). Adenomyosis as a disorder of the early and late human reproductive period. *Reproductive Medicine Online, 15(6),* 681-5. doi: 10.1016/s1472-6483(10)60535-4

Kwon, B., Ha, N., Jung, J., Kim, P.G., Kho, Y., Choi, K., & Ji, K. (2016). Effects of barium chloride exposure on hormones and genes of

363

the hypothalamic-pituitary-gonad axis, and reproduction of zebrafish (Danio rerio). *Bull Environ Contam Toxicol, 96(3)*, 341-6. doi: 10.1007/s00128-016-1731-9

Lee, K.H., Kim, J.K., Lee, M.A., Ko, Y.B., Yang, J.B., Kang, B.H., & Yoo, H.J. (2016). Relationship between uterine volume and discontinuation of treatment with levonorgestrel-releasing intrauterine devices in patients with adenomyosis. *Archives of Gynecology and Obstetrics, 294(3)*, 561-566. doi: 10.1007/s00404-016-4105-y

Lee, S.R., Yi, K.W., Song, J.Y., Seo, S.K., Lu, D.Y., Cho, S., & Kim, S.H. (2017). Efficacy and safety of long-term use of dienogest in women with ovarian endometrioma. *Reproductive Sciences, 25(3)*, 341-346. doi: 10.1177/1933719117725820

Lee, C. E., Yong, P.J., Williams, C., & Allaire, C. (2018). Factors associated with severity of irritable bowel syndrome symptoms in patients with endometriosis. *J Obstet Gynaecol Can, 40(2)*, 158-64. doi: 10.1016/j.jogc.2017.06.025

Leutner, M., Matzhold, C., Bellach, L., Deischinger, C., Harreiter, J., Thurner, S., Klimek, P., & Kautzky-Willer, A. (2019). Diagnosis of osteoporosis in statin-treated patients is dose-dependent. *Annals of the Rheumatic Diseases, 78(12)*. doi: 10.1136/annrheumdis-2019-215714

Liang, E. & Brown, B. (2021). Could it be Adenomyosis? The Bad Cousin of Endometriosis, An Unsuspected Cause of Heavy Painful Periods. Author Express, www.authorexpress.com

Lima, A.P., Moura, M.D., & Rosa eSilva, A.A.M. (2006). Prolactin and cortisol levels in women with endometriosis. *Brazilian Journal of Medical and Biological Research, 39(8)*, 1121-1127. doi:10.1590/s0100-879x2006000800015

Lipiski, E. (2000). Digestive Wellness. US:Keats Publishing

Mackoul, P. (2022). Advanced Fibroid Removal with the LAAM® Myomectomy. Retrieved from https:// innovativegyn.com/techniques/laam/

MacNamara, P., O'Shaughnessy, C., Manduca, P., & Loughrey, H.C. (1995). Progesterone receptors are expressed in human osteoblast-like cell lines and in primary human osteoblast cultures. *Calcified Tissue International, 57(6),* 436-444. doi: 10.1007/BF00301947

Malherbe, K., Khan, M., & Fatima, S. (2021). Fibrocystic Breast Disease. NCBI Bookshelf, Stat Pearls Publishing. Retrieved from ncbi.nlm.nih.gov/books/NBK551609/

Mamandi, M.M., Tu, K., VanWalraven, C., Austin, P.C., & Naylor, D.C. (2000). Postmenopausal estrogen replacement therapy and increased rates of cholecystectomy and appendectomy. *CMAJ, 162,* 1421-1424. Retrieved from https://www.ncbi.nlm.nih.gov/pmc/articles/ PMC1232454/

Mansukhani, N., Unni, J., Dua, M., Darbari, R., Malik, S., Verma, S., & Bathla, S. (2013). Are women satisfied when using levonorgestrel-releasing uterine system for treatment of abnormal uterine bleeding? *Journal of Mid-Life Health, 4(1),* 31-35. doi: 10.4103/0976-78--.109633

Maroun, P., Cooper, M.J., Reid, G.D., & Keirse, M.J. (2009). Relevance of gastrointestinal symptoms in endometriosis. *ANZJOG, 49(4),* 411-414. doi: 10.1111/j.1479-828X.2009.01030.x

Martin, M.B., Reiter, R., Pham, T., Avellanet, Y.R., Camara, J., Lahm, M., Pentecost, E., Pratap, K., Gilmore, B.A., Divekar, S., Dagata, R.S., Bull, J.L., & Stoica, A. (2003). Estrogen-like activity of metals n Mcf-7 breast cancer cells. *Endocrinology, 144(6),* 2425-2436. doi: 10.1210/en.2002-221054

Matalliotakis, I., Cakmak, H., Matalliotakis, M., Kappou, D., & Arici, A. (2012). High rate of allergies among women with endometriosis. *Journal of Obstetrics and Gynaecology, 32(3),* 291-293. doi: 10.3109/01443615.2011.644358

Mayani, A., Barel, S., Soback, S., & Almagor, M. (1997). Dioxin concentrations in women with endometriosis. *Human Reproduction, 12(2),* 373-5. doi: 10.1093/humrep/12.2.373

Mayo Clinic (2021). Fibrocystic Breasts. Retrieved from mayoclinic.org/diseases-conditions/fibrocystic-breasts/symptoms-causes/syc-20350438

Medici, N., Minucci, S., Nigro, V., Abbondanza, C., Armetta, I., Molinari, A.M., & Puca, G.A. (1989). Metal binding sites of the estradiol receptor from calf uterus and their possible role in the regulation of receptor function. *Biochemistry, 28(1),* 212-9. doi: 10.1021/ bio0427a029.

Mehdizadehkashi, A., Rokhgireh, S.,Tahermanesh, K., Eslahi, N., Minaeian, S., & Samimi, M. (2021). The effect of vitamin D supplementation on clinical symptoms and metabolic profiles in patients with endometriosis. *Gynecol Endocrinol, 37(7),* 640-645. doi: https://doi.org/10.1080/09513590.2021.1878138

Moore, J.S., Gibson, P.R., Perry, R.E., & Burgell, R.E. (2017). Endometriosis in patients with irritable bowel syndrome: Specific symptomatic and demographic profile, and response to the low FODMAP diet. *ANZJOG, 57(2),* 201-205. doi:10.1111/ajo.12594

Moore, R.W., Rudy, T.A., Lin, T.M., Ko, K., & Peterson, R.E. (2001). Abnormalities of sexual development in male rats with in utero and lactational exposure to the antiandrogenic plasticizer di(2-ethylhexyl) phthalate. *Environmental Health Perspectives, 109(3),* 229-237. doi: 10.1289/ehp.01109229

Moradi, M., Parker, M., Sneddon, A., Lopez, V., & Ellwood, D. (2019). The Endometriosis Impact Questionnaire (EIQ): A tool to measure the long-term impact of endometriosis on different aspects of women's lives. *BMC Womens Health, 19(1),* 64. doi: 10.1186/s12905-019-0762-x

Moraru I.G., Moraru A.G., Andrei M., Iordache, T., Drug, V., Diculescu, M., Portincasa, P. & Dumitrascu, D.L. (2014). Small intestinal bacterial overgrowth is associated to symptoms in irritable bowel syndrome: Evidence from a multicentre study in Romania. *Rom J Intern Med. 52(4),*143–150. Retrieved from https://pubmed.ncbi.nlm.nih.gov/ 25509557/

Moroshi, K., Yamamoto, H., Kamata, R., Shiraishi, F., Koda, T. & Morita, M. (2005). Estrogenic activity of 37 components of commercial sunscreen lotions evaluated by in vitro assays. *Journal of Toxicology in Vitro, (19)4,* 457-69. doi: 10.1016/j.tiv.2005.01.004

Nayyar, T., Bruner-Tran, K.L., Piestrzeniewicz-Ulanska, D. & Osteen, K.G. (2007). Developmental exposure of mice to TCDD elicits a similar uterine phenotype in adult animals as observed in women with endometriosis. *Reproductive Toxicology, 23(3),* 326-336. doi: 10.1016/j.reprotox.2006.09.007

Nezhat, C. (2021). Best Endometriosis Specialist in California. Retrieved from http://nezhat.org/endometriosis-treatment/endometriosis/

Nezhat, C. (2021). Diagnosing Bowel Endometriosis. Retrieved from http://nezhat.org/diagnosing-bowel-endometriosis-step-by-step-workup/

Nezhat, C. (2021). Endometriosis is a Whole-Body Disease. Retrieved from http://nezhat.org/endometriosis-treatment/history-of-endometriosis/

Novellas, S., Chassang, M., Delotte, J., Toullalan, O., Chevallier, A., Boouasis, J., & Chevalier, P. (2011). MRI characteristics of the uterine junctional zone: From normal to the diagnosis of adenomyosis. *American Journal of Roentgenology, 196(5),* 1206-13. doi: 10.2214/AJR.10.4877

Oiu, Y., Yuan, S., & Wang, H. (2020). Vitamin D status in endometriosis: a systematic review and meta-analysis. *Archives of Gynecology and Obstetrics, 302,* 141-152. doi: 10.1007/s00404-020-05576-5

Ota, H., Igarashi, S., Hatazawa, J., & Tanaka, T. (1998). Endothelial nitric oxide synthase in the endometrium during the menstrual cycle in patients with endometriosis and adenomyosis. *Fertility and Sterility, 69,* 303-308. Retrieved from http://www.ncbi.nlm.nih.gov/m/pubmed/9496346

Pageda, A.C., Bae, I.H., & Perkins, H.E. (1995). Review of 24 cases of uterine ablation failure. *Journal of Minimally Invasive Gynecology, 2(4),* 539. doi: 10.1016/S1074-3804(05)80588-2

Parikh, M., Maddaford, T., Austria, J.A., Aliani, M., Netticadan, T., & Pierce, G.N. (2019). Dietary flaxseed as a strategy for improving health. *Nutrients, 11(5),* 1171. doi.org/10.33990/nu11051171

Patel, B.G., Rudnicki, M., Yu, J., Shu, Y., & Taylor, R.N. (2017). Progesterone resistance in endometriosis: Origins, consequences, and interventions. *Acta Obstetricia et Gynecologica Scandinavica, 96(6),* 623-632. doi: 10.1111/aogs.13156

Paterni, I., Granchi, C., Katzenellenbogen, J. & Minutolo, F. (2014). Estrogen receptors alpha (ERα) and beta (ERβ): Subtype-selective ligands and clinical potential. *Steroids, 90,* 13-29. doi: 10.1016/j.steroids.2014.06.012

Pauwels, A., Schepens, P.J., D'Hooghe, T., Delbeke, L., Dhont, M., Brouwer, A., & Weyler, J. (2001). The risk of endometriosis and exposure to dioxins and polychlorinated biphenyls: A case-control study of infertile women. *Human Reproduction, 16(10),* 2050-5. doi: 10.1093/humrep/16.10.2050

Petrellluzzi, K.F., Garcia, M.C., Petta, C.A., Grassi-Kassisse, D.M., & Spadari-Bratfisch, R.C. (2008). Salivary cortisol concentrations, stress and quality of life in women with endometriosis and chronic pelvic pain. *Stress, 11(5),* 390-7. doi: 10.080/10253890701840610

Piazza, M. J. & Urbanetz, A. A. (2018). Environmental toxins and the impact of other endocrine disrupting chemicals in women's reproductive health. *JBRA Assisted Reproduction, 23(2),* 154-164. doi: 10.5935/1518-0557.20190016

Pop-Trajkovic, S., Popovic, J., Antic, V., Radovic, D., Stavanovic, M., & Vukomanovic, P. (2013). Stages of endometriosis: Does it affect in vitro fertilization outcome. *Taiwanese Journal of Obstetrics & Gynecology, 53(2),* 224-226. doi: 10.1016/j.tjog.2013.10.040

Porpora, M.G., Ingelido, A.M., DiDomenico, A., Ferro, A., Crobu, M., Pallate, D., Cardellli, M., Cosmi, E.V. & De Felip, E. (2006). Increased levels of polychlorobiphenyls in Italian women with endometriosis. *Chemosphere, 63(8),* 1361-1367. doi: 10.1016/j.chemosphere. 2005.09.022

Potera, C. (2006). Women's health: Endometriosis and PCB exposure. *Environmental Health Perspectives, 114(7),* A404. Retrieved from ncbi.nlm.nih.gov/pmc/articles/PMC1513298/

Quinones, M., Urrutia, R., Torres-Reveron, A., Vincent, K., & Flores, I. (2015). Anxiety, coping skills and hypothalamus-pituitary-adrenal

(HPA) axis in patients with endometriosis. *Journal of Reproductive Biology and Health, 3*: 2. doi: 10.7243/2054-0841-3-2

Reddy, B.S., Rozati, R., Reddy, B.V.R., & Raman, N.V. (2006). Association of phthalate esters with endometriosis in Indian women. *BJOG, 113(5),* 515-20. doi: 10.1111/j.1471-0528.200600925.x

Remorgida, V., Abbamonte, L.H., Ragni, N., Fulcheri, E., & Ferrero, S. (2007). Letrozole and desogestrel-only contraceptive pill for the treatment of stage IV endometriosis. *ANZJOG, 47,* 222-5. doi: 10.1111/j.1479-828X.2007.00722.x

Rice, K.M., Walker, E.M. Wu, M., Gillette, C., & Blough, E.R. (2014). Environmental mercury and its toxic effects. *Journal of Preventative Medicine and Public Health, 47(2),* 74-83. doi: 10.3961/jpmph.2014.47.2.74

Rier, S.E., Turner, W.E., Martin, D.C., Morris, R., Lucier, G.W., & Clark, G.C. (2001). Serum levels of TCDD and dioxin-like chemicals in Rhesus monkeys chronically exposed to dioxin: Correlation of increased serum PCB levels with endometriosis. *Toxicol Sci, 59(1),* 47-59. doi: 10.1093/toxsci/59.1/147

Riley, K. A., Davies, M.F., & Harkins, G. J. (2013). Characteristics of patients undergoing hysterectomy for failed endometrial ablation. *Journal of the Society of Laparoendoscopic Surgeons, 17(4),* 503-507. doi: 10.4293/108680813X13693422520602

Roby, R.R., Richardson, R.H., & Vojdani, A. (2006). Hormone allergy. *American Journal of Reproductive Immunology, 55,* 307-313. doi: 10.1111/j.1600-0897.2006.00373.x

Roman, H., Tuech, J.J., Juet, E., Bridoux, V., Khalil, H., Hennetier, C., Bubenheim, M., & Brinduse, L.A. (2019). Excision versus colorectal resection in deep endometriosis infiltrating the rectum: 5-year follow-up of patients enrolled in a randomized controlled trial. *Human Reproduction, 34(12),* 2362-2371. doi: 10.1093/humrep/dez217

Ruffo, G., Scopelliti, F., Manzoni, A., Sartori, A., Rossini, R., Ceccaroni, M., Minelli, L., Crippa, S., Partelli, S., & Falconi, M. (2014). Long-term outcome after laparoscopic bowel resections for deep infiltrating endometriosis: A single-center experience after 900 cases. *Biomed Res Int, 2014,* 463058. doi: 10.1155/2014/463058

Saidi, K., Sharma, S., & Ohlsson, B. (2020). A systematic review and meta-analysis of the associations between endometriosis and irritable bowel syndrome. *Eur J Obstet Gynecol Reprod Biol, 246,* 99-105. doi: 10.1016/j.ejogrb.2020.01.031

Salim, R., Riris, S., Saab, W., Abramov, B., Khadum, I., & Serhal, P. (2012). Adenomyosis reduces pregnancy rates in infertile women undergoing IVF. *Reproductive BioMedicine Online, 25(3),* 273-277. doi: 10.1016/j.rbmo.2012.05.003

Sasaki, K., Singh, A.C., Sulo, S., & Miller, C.E. (2014). Persistent bleeding after laparoscopic supracervical hysterectomy. *JSLS, 18(4),* e2014.002064. doi: 10.4293/JSLS.2014.002064

Sax, L. (2010). Polyethylene terephthalate may yield endocrine disruptors. *Environ Health Perspect, 118(4),* 445-448. doi: 10.1289/ehp.0901253

Schlumpf, M., Durrer, S., Faass, O., Ehnes, C., Fuetsch, M., Gaille, C., Henseler, M., Hofkamp, L., Maerkel, K., Reolon, S., Timms, B., Tresquerres, J.A. & Lichtensteiger, W. (2008). Developmental toxicity of UV filters and environmental exposure: A review. *International Journal of Andrology, 31(2),* 144-51. doi: 10.1111/j.1365-2605.2007.00856.x

Seckin, Tamer, M.D. (2021). A Letter from Dr. Seckin on Hysterectomies, Endometriosis, and Adenomyosis. Endometriosis Foundation of America. Retrieved from https:// endofound.org/a-letter-from-dr.-seckin-on-hysterectomies-endometriosis-vs-adenomyosis

Seckin, Tamer, MD. (2020). IBS is BS When it is Endometriosis...Culprit in the Misdiagnosis, and Years of Delay. Endometriosis Foundation of America. Retrieved from https://www.endofound.org/ibs-is-bs-when-it-is-endometriosis.culprit-in-the-misdiagnosis-and-years-of-delay-tamer-seckin-md

Seifert-Klauss, V. & Prior, J.C. (2010). Progesterone and bone: Actions promoting bone health in women. *J Osteoporos,* 845180. Retrieved from https://www.hindawi.com/journals/josteo

Seifert-Klauss, V., Schmidmayr, M., Hobmaier, E., & Wimmer, T. (2012). Progesterone and bone: a closer link than previously realized. *Climacteric, 15 (sup1),* 26-31. doi: 10.3109/13697137.2012.669530

Shah, S. (2012). Hormonal link to autoimmune allergies. *ISRN Allergy*, 910437. doi: 10.5402/2012/910437

Sheng, J., Zhang, W.Y., Zhang, J.P., & Lu, D. (2009). The LNS-IUS study on adenomyosis: A 3-year follow-up study on the efficacy and side effects of the use of levonorgestrel intrauterine system for the treatment of dysmenorrhea associated with adenomyosis. *Contraception, 79(3),* 189-93. doi: 10.1016/j.contraception.2008.11.004

Simsa, P., Mihalyi, A., Schoeters, G., Kippen, G., Kyama, C.M., Den Hond, E. M., Fulop, V., & D'Hooghe, T.M. (2010). Increased exposure to dioxin-like compounds is associated with endometriosis in a case-control study in women. *Reproductive Biomedicine Online, 20(5),* 681-8. doi: 10.1016/j.rbmo.2010.01.018

Sinaii, N., Cleary, S.D., Ballweg, M.L., Nieman, L.K., & Stratton, P. (2002). High rates of autoimmune and endocrine disorders, fibromyalgia, chronic fatigue syndrome and atopic diseases among women with endometriosis: A survey analysis. *Human Reproduction, 17(10),* 2715-2724. doi: https://doi.org/10.1093/humrep/17.10.2715

Sinervo, K. (2021). Adhesions: An Update. Retrieved from centerforendo.com/adhesions-update

Sinervo, K., Khan, Z., & Braverman, J. (2016). Infertility. Center for Endometriosis Care. Retrieved from https://centerforendo. com/infertility

Smith, M.P., Keay, S.D., Margo, F.C., Harlow, C.R., Wood, P.J., Cahill, D.J., & Hull, M.G.R. (2002). Total cortisol levels are reduced in the periovulatory follicle of infertile women with minimal-mild endometriosis. *American Journal of Reproductive Immunology, 47(1),* 52-56. doi:10.1034/j.1600-0897.2002.1o122.x

Smith, P.W. (2010). What You Must Know About Women's Hormones: Your Guide to Natural Hormone Treatments for PMS, Menopause, Osteoporosis, PCOS and More. US: Square One Publishers

Soysal, S., Soysal, M.E., Ozer, S., Gui, N. & Gezgin, T. (2004). The effects of post-surgical administration of goserelin plus anastrozole

371

compared to goserelin alone in patients with severe endometriosis: A prospective randomized trial. *Human Reproduction, 19(1),* 160. doi: 10.1093/humanrep/deh035

Stoica, A., Pentecost, E., & Martin, M.B. (2000). Effects of selenite on estrogen receptor α expression and activity in Mcf-7 breast cancer cells. *Journal of Cellular Biochemistry, 79(2),* 282-292. doi: 10.1002/1097-4644(20002 1101)79:2<282;;AID-JCB110>3.0.CO;2-V

Streuli, I., Dubuisson, J., Santulli, P., De Siegler, D., Batteux, F., & Chapron. C. (2014). An update on the pharmacological management of adenomyosis. *Expert Opinion on Pharmacotherapy, 15(16),* 2347-2360. doi: 10.1517/14656566.2014.953055

Su, P.H., Huang, P.C., Lin, C.Y., Ying, T.H., Chen, J.Y., & Wang, S.L. (2012). The effect of in utero exposure to dioxins and polychlorinated biphenyls on reproductive development in eight-year-old children. *Environ Int, 39(1),* 181-7. doi: 10.1016/j.envint.2011.09.009

Sydney Fibroid Clinic (2021). Why Endometrial Ablation for Adenomyosis Might Make Pain Worse? Retrieved from https://sydneyfibroidclinic.com.au/why-endometrial-ablation-for-adenomyosis-might-make-pain-worse

Sydney Fibroid Clinic (2021). Medical Therapy for Adenomyosis. Retrieved from https:// sydneyfibroidclinic.com.au/adenomyosis-treatments/medical-therapy/

Sydney Fibroid Clinic (2021). Mirena IUD for Adenomyosis. Retrieved from https://sydneyfibroidclinic.com.au/adenomyosis-treatments/mirena-iud/

Takaguchi, M. & Yoshihara, S. (2006). New aspects of cadmium as endocrine disruptor. *Environ Sci, 13(2),* 107-16. Retrieved from https://pubmed.ncbi.nlm.nih.gov/16788562/

Taran, F.A., Stewart, E.A. & Brucker, S. (2013). Adenomyosis: Epidemiology, risk factors, clinical phenotype and surgical and interventional alternatives to hysterectomy. *Geburtshife Frauenheilkd, 73(9),* 924-931. doi: 10.1055/s-0033-1350840

Tremellen, K. & Russell, P. (2011). Adenomyosis is a potential cause of recurrent implantation failure during IVF treatment. *ANZJOG, 51(3),* 280-283. doi:10.1111/j.1479-828X.2010.01276.x

Troisi, R., Hyer, M., Hatch, E.E., Titus-Ernstoff, L., Palmer, J.R., Strohsnitter, W.C., Herbst, A.L., Adam, E., & Hoover, R.N. (2013). Medical conditions among adult offspring prenatally exposed to diethylstilbestrol. *Epidemiology, 24(3),* 430-438. doi: 10.1097/EDE.0b013e318289bdf7

Untersmayr, E., Jensen, A.N., & Walch, K. (2017). Sex hormone allergy: Clinical aspects, causes and therapeutic strategies – update and secondary publication. *World Allergy Organ J, 10(1),* 45. doi: 10.1186/s40413-017-0176-x

Upson, K., DeRoos, A.J., Thompson, M.L., Sathyanarayana, S., Scholes, D., Barr, D.B. & Holt, V.L. (2013). Organochlorine pesticides and risk of endometriosis: Finding from a population-based case-control study. *Environmental Health Perspectives, 121,* 11-12. doi: 10.1289/ehp.1306648

Upson, K., Sathyanarayana, S., DeRoos, A.J., Thompson, M.L., Scholes, D., Dills, R. & Holt, V.L. (2013). Phthalates and risk of endometriosis. *Environ Res, 126,* 91-97. doi: 10.1016/envres.2013.07.003

UT Southwestern (2021). UT Southwestern Review Finds Hysterectomy can be Avoided for Common Gynecological Condition. Retrieved from utsouthwestern.edu/newsroom/articles/year-2021/hysterectomy-gynecological-condition.html

Vannuccini, S., Clemenza, S., Rossi, M., & Petraglia, F. (2021). Hormonal treatments for endometriosis: The endocrine background. *Rev Endocr Metab Disorder, 23(3),* 333-355 doi: 10.1007/s11154-021-09666-w

Veloso, H.G. (2022). FODMAP Diet: What You Need to Know. Johns Hopkins Medicine. Retrieved from www.hopkinsmedicine.org/health/wellness-and-prevention/fodmap-diet-what-you-need-to-know

Vercellini, P., Consonni, D., Dridi, D., Bracco, B., Frattaruolo, M.P., & Somigliana, E. (2014). Uterine adenomyosis and in vitro fertilization outcome: A systematic review and meta-analysis. *Human Reproduction, 29(5),* 964-977. doi: 10.1093/humrep/deu041

Vercellini, P., Pietropaolo, G., DeGiorgi, O., Pasin, R., Chiodini, A., & Crosignani, P.G. (2005). Treatment of symptomatic rectovaginal endometriosis with an estrogen-progestogen combination versus low-dose norethindrone acetate. *Fertility and Sterility, 84,* 1375-87. doi: 10.1016/j.fertnstert.2005.03.083

Vercellini,P., Somigliana, E., Buggio, L., Giussy, B., Frattaruolo, M.P., & Fedele, L. (2012). "I can't get no satisfaction": Deep dyspareunia and sexual functioning in women with rectovaginal endometriosis. *Fertility and Sterility, 98(6),* 1503-1511. doi: 10.1016/j.fertnstert.2012.07.1129

Walsh (2011). Study: Even 'BPA-free' plastics leach endocrine-disrupting chemicals. *Time.* Retrieved 14 September 2016.

Women's Health. (2021). Think You Have Adenomyosis? This Might Help. Retrieved from womenshealth.com.au/think-you-have-adenomyosis-this-might-help/

Wu, Y., Strawn, E., Basir, Z., Halverson, G., & Guo, S.W. (2006). Promoter hypermethylation of progesterone receptor isoform B (PRB) in endometriosis. *Epigenetics, 1(2),* 106-11. doi: 10.4161/epi.1.2.2766

Yang, J.Z., Agarwal, S.K., & Foster, W.G. (2000). Subchronic exposure to 2,3,7,8-tetracholodibenzo-p-dioxin modulates the pathophysiology of endometriosis in the cynomolgus monkey. *Toxicol Sci, 56(2),* 374-81. doi: 10.1093/toxsci/56.2.374

Yeung, P., Sinervo, K., Winer, W., & Albee, R.B. (2011). Complete laparoscopic excision of endometriosis in teenagers: Is post operative hormonal suppression necessary? *Fertility and Sterility, 95(6),* 1909-12. doi: 10.1016/j.fertnstert.2011.02.037

Yuk, J.S., Shin, J.S., Shin, J.Y., Oh, E., Kim, H., & Park, W.I. (2015). Nickel allergy is a risk factor for endometriosis: An 11-year population-based nested case-control study. *PLoS One, 10(10),* e0139388. doi: 10.1371/journal.pone.0139388

Zhu, B., Chen, Y., Shen, X., Liu, X., & Guo, S.W. (2016). Anti-platelet therapy hold promise in treating adenomyosis: Experimental evidence. *Reprod Biol Endocrinol, 14(1),* 66. doi: 10.1186/s12958-016-0198-1

Index

B

C

F

J

L

M

U

V

W

X

Y

Z

About the Author

Maria Yeager has a B.S. in Microbiology and is certified as a Cytogenetic Technologist through the American Society of Clinical Pathology (ASCP). She has twenty years of laboratory experience working at places such as Quest Diagnostics and The University of Texas Health Science Center at San Antonio (UTHSCSA). She also has a M.S. degree in Holistic Nutrition and a Family Herbalist certificate. She dealt with adenomyosis for seventeen years before obtaining an official diagnosis only after hysterectomy. She has authored multiple books on adenomyosis including Adenomyosis: A Significantly Neglected and Misunderstood Uterine Disorder, Why Can't Anyone Help Me? The Nightmare of Adenomyosis, and Adenomyosis: The Women Speak. All books are available on Amazon. Maria currently resides in Virginia.

www.ingramcontent.com/pod-product-compliance
Lightning Source LLC
Chambersburg PA
CBHW051945150726
47999CB00004B/1253